DEVELOPING SUPPORT GROUPS
FOR INDIVIDUALS WITH
EARLY-STAGE ALZHEIMER'S DISEASE

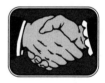

DEVELOPING SUPPORT GROUPS FOR INDIVIDUALS WITH EARLY-STAGE ALZHEIMER'S DISEASE
Planning, Implementation, and Evaluation

by

Robyn Yale, L.C.S.W.
Project Specialist in
Aging and Alzheimer's Disease
San Francisco, California

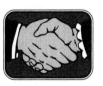

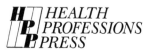
HEALTH
PROFESSIONS
PRESS

Baltimore • London • Winnipeg • Sydney

Health Professions Press
Post Office Box 10624
Baltimore, Maryland 21285-0624

Typeset by Signature Typesetting & Design, Baltimore, Maryland.
Manufactured in the United States of America by
The Maple Press Company, York, Pennsylvania.

First printing, November 1995
Second printing, February 1998

Library of Congress Cataloging-in-Publication Data
Yale, Robyn.
   Developing support groups for individuals with early-stage
   Alzheimer's disease : planning, implementation, and evaluation / by
   Robyn Yale.
      p.   cm.
   Includes bibliographical references and index.
   ISBN 1-878812-26-2
      1. Alzheimer's disease—Patients—Counseling of.   2. Self-help
   groups.   3. Alzheimer's disease—Patients—Social networks.
   I. Title.
   RC523.Y35   1995
   362.1'96831—dc20   95-6672
                                                              CIP

British Library Cataloguing-in-Publication data are available from the
British Library.

CONTENTS

FOREWORD

It is my pleasure to recommend *Developing Support Groups for Individuals with Early-Stage Alzheimer's Disease: Planning, Implementation, and Evaluation.* This excellent reference is the only one of its kind to be based on sound clinical experience and to be written by someone with expertise in this specialized intervention. The book is also unique in that it integrates the three distinct components—research, practice, and training—demonstrating a well-rounded, clearly delineated, and comprehensive approach.

The concept of support services for individuals with Alzheimer's disease is still relatively new but has become recognized as a major area of unmet need in the field. As a result, the underpinnings of a new structural foundation have been developed. It is, however, crucial that we continue to make an effort to expand our understanding of what people with Alzheimer's disease experience and what is most helpful to them in coping with the illness. Expansion of programs, policy, research, education, and outreach efforts specific to the early or beginning stages of the disease are not only important, but are urgently needed. Providers of dementia care are reaching out in greater numbers for ideas about how best to respond to the people in their regions who have early-stage Alzheimer's disease and are seeking information and support about their condition.

Robyn Yale has been one of only a few pioneers to call attention to these issues and work to create a new service infrastructure. She has had the vision and capability to collaborate with the Alzheimer's Association and other key organizations to promote public and professional awareness about people with Alzheimer's disease. Her support group model has been a major prototype for early-stage Alzheimer's disease programs developed across and outside of the United States. The tools she constructed have been carefully assembled herein so that others may use them to craft similar successes.

Developing Support Groups for Individuals with Early-Stage Alzheimer's Disease: Planning, Implementation, and Evaluation provides user-friendly materials and guidelines for setting up, conducting, and administering these groups. Chapters 1–7 walk the reader through a systematic process in a step-by-step manner, articulate critical challenges, and offer recommendations in regard to each decision point that may be encountered along the way. Procedures suggested for screening and enrolling group participants, observing and evaluating group sessions, and providing publicity and outreach are among those explained. Ready-to-use sample forms are also included. Chapter 8 contains realistic role-play exercises that can be part of consultation with colleagues or supervision to train support group facilitators. Chapter 9 documents the results of a research study that brings to life the experiences of group participants and their family members' interesting reactions. All told, this engaging book is thorough, well written, and relevant to a wide audience of health professionals, academicians, agency board members and administrators, care providers, and program planners.

Perhaps most importantly, readers of this book will be given the courage and skills to accept the challenge of working with individuals who have early-stage Alzheimer's disease. With this book in hand, practitioners will be taken by the hand, encouraged, and led through the development of a support group intervention. This volume makes a valuable contribution not only by offering specific information, but also by instilling in others the courage to use this information.

Rea Kahn, R.N., M.P.S.
Support Group Coordinator
Alzheimer's Association
New York City Chapter

PREFACE

"It helps to know you aren't alone—listening to how others deal with similar problems ... it makes me feel much better to know that there are people like me."

This statement speaks of the power that support groups have to assist people in coping with specific difficulties. The statement could be describing a group focused on, for example, surviving cancer, abstaining from alcohol, or caring for a relative with a chronic illness. It was made, however, by someone in a group for individuals with early-stage Alzheimer's disease. These were individuals *of all ages* who were seeking information and support while they had only mild impairment as a result of Alzheimer's disease.

The mental health needs of people with early dementia, which are unique and newly recognized, have been seriously overlooked and underserved. As early detection methods improve and concerns mount about incidence, costs, and consequences of the disease, this gap in the continuum of dementia care has become glaringly apparent. The distinctiveness of the early stages of Alzheimer's disease and the lack of programs targeting people with the disease are, though, finally coming into public focus.

The potential benefits of support groups for people who have been told their diagnoses while in the early stages of dementia have just begun to be explored. Ramifications of this new direction are particularly important as other viable treatment options remain elusive.

This book is intended to be a stepping stone in making support services for individuals with Alzheimer's disease more widely available. It synthesizes my research, clinical, and training experience, which includes the following:

1. A manual I wrote entitled *A Guide to Facilitating Support Groups for Newly Diagnosed Alzheimer's Patients*, published in 1991 by the Greater San Francisco Bay Area Chapter of the Alzheimer's Association, which provided a frame of reference and general guidelines for this model

2. A Pilot Research Grant from the National Alzheimer's Association to the University of California, San Francisco, in 1992, which studied the responses of individuals with early dementia and their responses to the illness and to this support group intervention

3. A regional workshop, cosponsored by the Bay Area and Marin County Chapters of the Alzheimer's Association, which was held in 1993 (Materials developed for this workshop formed the basis for this book and many other training forums.)

An overview of the approach and terms used herein can be found in the Introduction. Briefly, the support group model delineated in this book utilizes a discussion format to offer a combination of education, emotional support, and practical assistance. Because of the intensity of issues and feelings generated, these groups must be led by facilitators who have solid credentials and are appropriately supervised.

The advantage of this model is that it is low cost and requires relatively few resources (e.g., space, supplies) to implement. Furthermore, its fundamental underpinning is that people with early dementia who want assistance will find the support group to be a safe place to deal with reactions to their condition. And, while anguish is to be expected, it is also constructive to explore and build on the therapeutic dimensions of wellness and vitality. These concepts can be cornerstones in the foundation of a new service infrastructure.

The approach outlined herein is by no means the only option. There are other models, including support groups in which individuals with early dementia and their family members participate together, "clubs" that offer therapeutic activities and outings appropriate for people with mild dementia, and programs that provide the participants community volunteer and/or vocational opportunities. These efforts are applauded, and more information about them would be welcome!

The truth is that no one approach is suitable for all individuals with Alzheimer's disease. For example, some people who inquire about a support group may have too much cognitive impairment to participate in the program but also function at a higher level than individuals in dementia-specific adult day care centers. These people might be perfect for an activity-oriented "club." Some people whose first inquiry is directed to an activity program might actually be seeking meaningful work of some kind. Each person with Alzheimer's disease should be assessed for participation in any program based on his or her individual personality, coping style, abilities, and preferences, rather than on stereotyped assumptions and misperceptions.

My vision is one in which the entire continuum of dementia care is even more diversified, beginning earlier (e.g., prediagnostic information and counseling) and ending later (e.g., postplacement and bereavement counseling). The range of service options would correspond to the *gradations* of need within and between the commonly recognized stages (i.e., early, middle, and late). Connection and continuity among these services would also be strengthened for ease of referral and follow-up.

Of course, the ultimate goal is the eradication of Alzheimer's disease. Fortunately, with all the attention and scientific expertise dedicated to the disease, there is great promise and hope. In the interim, however, these individuals — just like those with any other terminal illness—must be allowed to retain and nurture that which makes them uniquely human. We must meet them with our eyes and hearts wide open, allowing them to grasp and participate in the full spectrum of care and life to which they are entitled.

The process of educating ourselves and each other to further this aim can occur through ongoing pooling and exchange of knowledge and resources. Information and support is as crucial to professionals as it is to the individuals with Alzheimer's disease in this new endeavor. Directions to pursue include the following:

- Work with local colleagues (e.g., health care providers, caregiver support group leaders) to facilitate recognition and referral of people with early-stage Alzheimer's disease to new services.

- Evaluate new programs you develop through ongoing research and clinical documentation. Consider collaboration with multisite centers to increase the scope and power of studies that can be done.

- Work with policy makers to advocate for the expansion of dementia-care services and more responsiveness to individuals with early-stage Alzheimer's disease and their families.

- Collaborate with local, national, and international organizations to coordinate information on early dementia and relevant services.

- Provide the lay and professional public with educational material and events targeted toward early dementia so that individuals with Alzheimer's disease and their families who are not yet connected to services can see themselves in positive images and learn what is available to them.

Because these goals are quite ambitious, this book has been written to accommodate a cross section of readers, including clinicians, researchers, service providers, and administrators. The intent is to conceptualize and systematize this particular model in hope of making it tangible and motivating others to expand services for individuals with early dementia and their families.

Groups may be conducted by private practitioners or under auspices of some kind; many configurations are possible. Therefore, the ideas presented here are addressed to you, the reader, whether you are the potential facilitator, a program planner, staff in an agency sponsoring a group, a funder, or a person curious or connected in some other way.

My hope in writing this book is to demystify the process of talking with people about having Alzheimer's disease and bring forward hope and optimism. Perhaps you will become inspired or encouraged to develop a program for individuals with early dementia in your community. At the very least, you may become a bit more convinced of the possibilities and a bit less frightened by a vague sense of foreboding or mystery. After all, those who work in the dementia-care field must be at least as courageous as those who are served by it.

As Goethe said,

Knowing is not enough; we must act.
Willing is not enough; we must do.

Please feel free to contact me if you would like to correspond about your own experience; connect with others specializing in this area; or receive further research, training, or practice information. Additional education materials available include an international newsletter and fact sheets on early dementia.

Robyn Yale, L.C.S.W.
Specialized Alzheimer's Projects and Services
1067 Filbert Street, Suite 100
San Francisco, California 94133
Telephone and fax: (415) 673-3881

ACKNOWLEDGMENTS

Sincere thanks and deep appreciation are extended to those who have either directly or indirectly supported my professional efforts.

The Alzheimer's Association
      Greater San Francisco Bay Area
      and Marin County Chapters
            for funding to compile a portion of these
            materials

The Alzheimer's Association, National Office
      for research funding

Joseph Barbaccia, M.D.
      University of California, San Francisco
      Medical Center
            for giving credence, opportunity, and prudent
            guidance

ACKNOWLEDGMENTS

Linda Mitteness, Ph.D.
    University of California, San Francisco
    Medical Center
        for technical expertise and assistance

Catherine Lee, M.A.
        for invaluable perceptiveness and support

David Assmann, my husband
        for design, production, consultation, and
        tenacious encouragement

*For the individuals with Alzheimer's disease
and their families who so courageously opened
their hearts in pioneering this work—
providing new and extraordinary information
to the field of Alzheimer's research*

May their voices be heard and heeded!

DEVELOPING SUPPORT GROUPS FOR INDIVIDUALS WITH EARLY-STAGE ALZHEIMER'S DISEASE

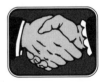

INTRODUCTION

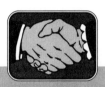

- Conceptualizing the challenge
- Theoretical background
- Explanation of terms
- A growing movement
- How to use this book

CONCEPTUALIZING THE CHALLENGE

"I'd like people to know—I have a lot of life left..."

The voice of this research study participant conveys a compelling message. Early-stage dementia is characterized not only by impairments that have become perceptible, but by abilities remaining intact as well. Each person responds differently to the dawning awareness of difficulties and newly required adjustments. Although some people cope by denying their condition, others display an amazing resilience and determination as they face the illness.

A major "blind spot" in the field of dementia care has categorically denied most people with Alzheimer's disease any opportunity to react and to strategize in regard to their condition. In many cases, those who have the illness are not even told of their diagnosis by clinicians, service providers, or family members. Although this may be appropriate in instances where an individual has too much cognitive impairment or resistance, or is too distraught to process medical information, it does not hold true for those who are concerned about what is wrong and want to better understand and cope with the illness.

An in-depth analysis of the pros and cons of telling people their diagnosis is beyond the scope of this book. Chapter 1 discusses this issue briefly. The crucial point here is that inroads must be made whereby individuals with early-stage Alzheimer's disease who seek assistance can receive it in order to deal with their emotional reactions, problem-solve their current situations, and plan for the future.

Chapters 1–8 attempt to lay some of this groundwork by providing information on developing a specific program model for a very specific subpopulation. This type of support group is not right for everyone, and selecting participants and facilitators for it should be done with great care. Equally clear, though, is the fact that growing numbers of skilled and dedicated service providers are recognizing an increasing demand in this area and are responding to requests for help in a variety of ways, thereby changing the face of the current infrastructure.

Some of these professionals have modestly described a sensation of "flying by the seat of their pants" in trying out new interventions. Yet, feedback from clients and colleagues has been very positive and so their efforts continue. Following their instincts and the blueprint mapped while listening closely to individuals with early-stage Alzheimer's disease, they are learning as they go along and experiencing the challenges and rewards of working with this interesting population.

Although venturing into unfamiliar territory can be a little unsettling, perhaps readers of this book will decide to do it too. Many of the principles a facilitator of this type of support group would use are similar to those used in other support group situations and other dementia-care settings, such as day programs, residential facilities, and information and referral centers. Specialized credentials and training recommended particularly for facilitators of this group are discussed in Chapter 3, and distinctive group dynamics and techniques are found in Chapter 5.

THEORETICAL BACKGROUND

Although relatively few have written about support groups for individuals with dementia in the literature, new service efforts can and should be built on a sound theoretical foundation. The reader is referred to Yale (1991) for further information on the background and context of this intervention.

Much of the research on Alzheimer's disease up to 1995 has focused on the impact of stress upon family caregivers, especially in regard to the individual's cognitive and functional status. Limited research has been aimed at understanding the perceptions and experiences of those who have dementia. Although individuals with moderate-to-severe impairment are generally less able to articulate their thoughts and feelings, many who have only mild impairment *can* identify and address their concerns about the illness.

Depression is a common reaction to the losses that accompany major developmental tasks and crises. Multiple changes in abilities, roles, and relationships may occur as a natural part of the aging process and can be traumatic when compounded by a chronic, debilitating illness. A significant proportion of those diagnosed with dementia have additional symptoms associated with major depression. And, cognitive decline may be exacerbated by depression—as well as by some of the medications used to treat it.

The "experts" have diverse opinions about whether depression in people with Alzheimer's disease is a result of facing the reality of having the illness or from lacking an opportunity to do so when excluded from conversations about it. Numerous other theories concerning factors contributing to depression also exist (e.g., biochemistry, physical health, support systems), which means that the answer is not at all clear-cut. In fact, just as there are many people who have Alzheimer's disease, there are many different explanations for it, and understanding the circumstances of each requires independent exploration.

However, psychotherapeutic interventions have typically been discounted on the assumption that individuals with Alzheimer's disease are unable to acknowledge and express their emotions. The basic clinical goals are, though, the following:

- Establishing rapport
- Fostering fulfilling interpersonal relationships
- Facilitating grief work and coming to terms with new circumstances

A point beyond acceptance has even been conceptualized whereby a loss is finally reformulated into a challenge for growth, resulting in a new attitude toward living with the "strength to carry on." Although this process has not been documented in people with Alzheimer's disease, the possibility of each having (and working through) an individualized grief reaction cannot be discarded.

Support groups have been effective in helping people deal with a range of difficulties and life transitions. Various types of groups exist and diverse theoretical orientations guide their structure and format. Often, the nature of the group process is such that the constructive "give and take" that occurs among people with common problems becomes nurturing and healing in itself.

Support groups that combine education and emotional expression are widely available to family members of people with Alzheimer's disease. Potential benefits include a better understanding of the illness, decreased isolation, attention to future planning, and an emphasis on self-care for the caregiver. There is no reason to assume that individuals with Alzheimer's disease do not have analogous needs for connection with and affirmation by others, as well as needs for practical assistance. In fact, involvement in usual work, social, and leisure activities must often be curtailed relatively early in the disease course. Support groups can provide a therapeutic environment for the participants in which changes in lifestyle may be openly discussed, information and reassurance about symptoms offered, and community resources to assist with problem solving identified.

Participation of people with Alzheimer's disease in support groups may secondarily benefit their caregivers if their mental health does indeed improve. Furthermore, open discussion about the illness in a support group may stimulate communication about important matters at home, allowing for emotional exchange and appropriate involvement by the person with the disease in health care, legal, and financial planning decisions. This in turn could lead to early utilization of such other services as family therapy and legal consultation.

Although knowledge about Alzheimer's disease proliferated in the 1980s and 1990s, most of the literature and services available have focused on the long-term implications of the illness, rather than on its beginning stages. Adult day care has traditionally served the individual with moderate-to-severe Alzheimer's disease, leaving a large gap in follow-up for those who have only mild impairment at the time of diagnostic evaluation. Few caregiver support groups or educational materials deal specifically with early dementia. However, a great deal of research has reported that the well-being of most caregivers is jeopardized because they do not receive help for many years.

As overall estimates of the prevalence of Alzheimer's disease continue to rise and more individuals are diagnosed while in the early stages, it is imperative that more services targeting this point in the disease course be developed. Costs in terms of economics, health, and quality of life will be much higher in the long run if these unmet needs continue to be ignored. This book outlines an intervention that seeks to redress the lack of attention to those people who have Alzheimer's disease and to the issues that make the beginning stages of the illness unique for these individuals and their caregivers.

EXPLANATION OF TERMS

As service providers for dementia-related illnesses begin to focus on individuals with early-stage Alzheimer's disease, many different phrases are being used in reference to this population. Various approaches and types of programs are being discussed, and little standardization has been imposed during this exciting time of exploration. However, confusion often results when terms that are not synonymous are used interchangeably. It is important, therefore, to clarify mixed meanings and reduce potential misunderstandings in communication. Ultimately, this will require a collaborative effort to establish a common language. Explanations of the terms used in this book are offered below to begin this process:

- *Early Stage*—Clinicians often use the terms early-, middle-, and late-stage Alzheimer's disease to describe approximate points in the progression of the disease course. The increasing degree of impairment over time is correspondingly characterized as mild, moderate, or severe. These distinctions are somewhat imprecise and overlapping (e.g., "early-to-middle stage," "moderate-to-severe impairment"). Although there is a good deal of variability in the definitions and measures ascribed to each category, certain generalizations can be made.

Early-stage Alzheimer's disease is one way to identify individuals (of any age) who have only mild impairment due to symptoms of dementia. For example, little assistance is initially needed with self-care activities. Gradually (often slowly and barely noticeably), confusion and forgetfulness become apparent as cognitive and functional abilities are increasingly affected by the illness. Many individuals in the early stages of Alzheimer's disease are aware of and concerned about these changes, unlike individuals in the later stages, whose capacities for introspection and comprehension are compromised.

There are certain behaviors that caregivers must cope with that also tend to correlate to the individual's stage or level of impairment. For instance, repetitive questions and word-finding problems are common in the early stages of dementia, while wandering or inability to recognize others indicates more severe impairment. Caregivers of people with early-stage Alzheimer's disease may be newly learning about the disease and the service system, and struggling with such decisions as whether the individuals should continue to drive or live alone. As the disease progresses, of course, more care and supervision are required in all areas of daily life.

Neither age nor recency of diagnosis are predictive of a person's stage or level of impairment. Both younger and older people with mild dementia are equally faced with emotional adjustments and disruptions in identity, lifestyle, and relationships. Experience has also shown that those of different ages can relate quite well to one another in a support group focused on talking about and coping with Alzheimer's disease.

Although ultimately it may be desirable to diversify program options based on specialized needs, it should not be claimed that one subgroup of people with Alzheimer's disease is more worthy of services than another. No individual's longevity or rate of disease progression can be predicted, so younger *and* older people with early-stage Alzheimer's disease may have many years of good health, high functioning, and life left ahead of them, or they may (unfortunately) not. Thus, this book advocates that a first step is to have more services for people of all ages with early-stage Alzheimer's disease become more widely available.

How then can someone determine who is appropriate for the support group described? Each individual's level of impairment should be assessed along with other specific criteria that are detailed in Chapter 1.

- *Newly Diagnosed*—This term was previously used with the assumption that people who have newly received a diagnosis of Alzheimer's disease are likely to be in the early stages of the illness (i.e., have only mild impairment). Technically, though, it actually refers to the *recency* of diagnosis and is not predictive of the severity of symptoms. That is, some individuals do not seek diagnostic evaluation until they already have severe impairment, and others may remain with only mild impairment for quite some time after they are diagnosed. Thus, a person's cognitive status is more accurately described by the stage (early, middle, or late) or level of impairment (mild, moderate, or severe) than by the amount of time since his or her diagnosis.

- *Early Onset*—This term, sometimes used synonymously with *young onset*, refers to people who are younger when their symptoms of dementia first begin. There is no uniformly recognized age at which the onset of disease is considered "early." For instance, some may think of the early 60s as young, while others consider that to be an older age. In addition, it is becoming less common for all people to retire at a designated age; some choose to do so way before and some way after the previous markers of 62 or 65 years of age. According to the *Diagnostic and Statistical Manual of Mental Disorders* (4th ed.) (American Psychiatric Association, 1994), the criteria for early-onset Alzheimer's disease include being 65 years old or younger. But in the world of practice, individual programs (e.g., regional Alzheimer's Association chapters) each determine their own cut-off age for membership in an early-onset support group.

In scientific research, efforts are proceeding to determine whether the cause and course of Alzheimer's disease are different for those whose illness strikes, for example, during their 40s and 50s from that for those in their 80s. In addition, some support group leaders believe that younger people with Alzheimer's disease have different issues from those of older people with Alzheimer's disease because of where they are in the life span. However, it is important to determine each person's needs on an individual basis and to beware of overgeneralizing about the relationship between age and the effect the illness has on life circumstances.

There are two other terms frequently used to characterize this population. One is *early dementia,* often used synonymously with the term *mild dementia,* indicating the presence of minimal cognitive and functional impairment due to Alzheimer's disease. *Early dementia* is also a general way to refer to the beginning point in the illness, which is when symptoms are relatively mild.

The other term often used is *early diagnosed*, which is technically incorrect. Because the word "early" is now used both in the contexts of age *and* severity of illness, it is important to specify its meaning. For some, early diagnosed refers to people who are diagnosed with Alzheimer's disease while they are relatively young. As discussed above, *early onset* would be the more appropriate term here. For others, *early diagnosed* refers to people who are diagnosed while in the early stages of Alzheimer's disease (i.e., with only mild impairment). In this regard, *early stage* would be more accurate.

A controversial and important question is often raised about the model described in this book. Is it *therapy*, or is it a *support group?* Often, the divergence of styles and approaches used in support groups blurs these semantic distinctions. For example, traditional group psychotherapy in inpatient or outpatient settings is facilitated by a professional therapist who delves deeply into the participants' difficulties (around a particular issue or illness) and seeks to relate maladaptive coping mechanisms to life conflicts. Support groups, however, are led by both professional therapists and laypersons experienced with the issue of focus and typically combine education, emotional support, and practical assistance.

However, some support groups, including the one described in this book, use a blend of supportive and psychotherapeutic techniques. The power of the group process, harnessed through relationships among the facilitator and participants, can be similarly activated by both techniques. People with Alzheimer's disease discuss traumatic changes and feelings related to the illness. They also empathize with one another, share coping strategies, and focus on strengths in the group. This may be considered to have therapeutic effects even if it is not called "therapy."

12

There has been concern and consensus expressed in the Alzheimer's disease field that support groups for people with Alzheimer's disease should be implemented only by professionals who are trained to deal with intense discussions and emotional reactions. This is one level at which differentiation of labels certainly makes sense. Even so, what is important is that the facilitator respond to what comes up in each meeting and handle it accordingly in ways that may vary by group session, mood, membership, and the leader's own style.

The format of the support group for people with early-stage Alzheimer's disease is described further in Chapter 5.

The term *group facilitator* is used interchangeably in this book with *group leader*. As mentioned previously, there are many types of support groups that are led by people with different backgrounds. The support group for people with Alzheimer's disease should be run and/or closely supervised by a professional therapist who has specific credentials and additional training as recommended in Chapter 3. Information in the book that is geared toward the *facilitator* but addresses administrative issues may also apply to such readers as agency staff or board members and program planners.

Because it is used so frequently in this manual, the term *group* is occasionally replaced with *program* or *service.*

The term *individual with Alzheimer's disease* is used interchangeably with [support group] *participant* in this book. The word *patient* is used in the research reported in Chapter 9. This is not meant to be depersonalizing, but is used in the context of someone who has been diagnosed with a medical condition and is receiving ongoing evaluation and care. In addition, *family member* is occasionally used synonymously with *caregiver.* It is recognized, though, that not all caregivers are related to the people with Alzheimer's disease with whom they are involved, and not all family members can be considered caregivers.

A GROWING MOVEMENT

The absence of standardized terminology around early dementia underscores the newness of this whole area. Although the clinical rationale for support groups for individuals with Alzheimer's disease has been apparent to the few professionals who have experienced it since the mid-1980s, little systematic research has been reported. The study documented in Chapter 9 is a beginning attempt to describe the group process and demonstrate the feasibility of this intervention. The findings that follow echo and strengthen the foundation for new services:

- Caregivers reported that the participants' mood and self-esteem improved as a result of the support group experience.
- The participants looked forward to attending meetings and felt less isolated and more understood.
- After participating in the support group, the individuals tended to seek information about other dementia-related services (e.g., day programs, counseling).

Awareness and interest in the person with Alzheimer's disease on the part of organizations that focus on the illness has grown tremendously in the 1990s. Support groups have been started by clinicians in private practice and in such settings as day programs, residential facilities, and mental health centers in the United States as well as in other countries. A network is slowly but surely forming to inform, support, and connect involved service providers.

However, there is still so much more to be done. As of 1994, only approximately 30 out of 221 local chapters of the National Alzheimer's Association have begun early-stage Alzheimer's disease programs, according to the Association's Patient and Family Services Department. Although that is an impressive start, it leaves many regions undeveloped in regard to services for people with Alzheimer's disease. In fairness, it has been necessary for the Alzheimer's Association to take some time to reexamine its mission and policies because it has been primarily a grass roots organization focused on family, rather than on support for the people with Alzheimer's disease. In the meantime, then, efforts must proceed outside of and in collaboration with the Alzheimer's Association as well.

Every month or so, an exciting biomedical research finding is reported in the news media. For example, the detection of Alzheimer's disease may someday be possible through a skin, eye, or genetic test. Each new discovery brings hope of an eventual cure for Alzheimer's disease, but also portends that the need to offer support services to those who learn they have the disease will continue to be urgent and ever-increasing.

As the need for more services is recognized and support groups become known as viable and vital to people with Alzheimer's disease as well as to their caregivers, this option must be made more widely available.

HOW TO USE THIS BOOK

This book discusses, then, the "nuts and bolts" of setting up, conducting, and overseeing a support group for people with early-stage Alzheimer's disease. The materials offered in this book are adapted from the research study described in Chapter 9 for use in practice settings. It is important to stress that these sample forms are not revised with data collection for research purposes in mind, although they may offer a good basis for that. **All the sample forms provided are reproducible and available to copy and use as long as credit is given to the author. Please note that only the *forms* in this book may be reproduced without obtaining prior written permission from the author.**

The recommendations sequentially provided in this book are suggestions only and should be thought of as guidelines for each reader's own journey. There are no definitive answers because of the newness of this area and the fact that the decisions made will ultimately depend on each individual's situation, setting, and style.

1

ESTABLISHING CRITERIA FOR GROUP PARTICIPATION

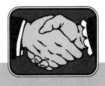

- Multifaceted selection criteria
- Level and assessment of cognitive functioning
- Obtaining and reviewing medical records
- Other dementia-related diagnoses
- Willingness to acknowledge and discuss the illness

The key to a successful support group for individuals with early-stage Alzheimer's disease is careful identification of the characteristics that define participants as appropriate for the group. First among many planning decisions to be made, then, are the guidelines by which the group facilitator will select the right group members from the many who may want to be involved. This chapter addresses the establishment of these guidelines.

MULTIFACETED SELECTION CRITERIA

An important preliminary step is making clear decisions about the desired characteristics of the participants for the group. Once these are identified, group members can be selected in a consistent and systematic manner. It is likely that individuals who have only mild cognitive impairment, who have communication and social skills appropriate for the group setting, and who are open about their condition will be most able to discuss their concerns about Alzheimer's disease and will value the chance to do so.

Many of the guidelines below describe early (rather than middle- or late-stage) symptoms of dementia. Other recommendations are offered for consideration in further delineating the target population.

- The individual has a diagnosis of probable Alzheimer's disease (or a related disorder) documented by a physician or geriatric assessment clinic professional.

- The individual was told about the diagnosis (by a medical doctor or family member) and at least occasionally acknowledges memory loss or confusion.
- The individual has early dementia as evidenced by mild cognitive impairment upon testing and interviewing.
- The individual has relatively intact communication skills, such as the ability to sustain conversation, express him- or herself, and comprehend others despite difficulty with word finding or speech.
- The individual is able and willing to discuss feelings and experiences related to the illness.
- The individual is appropriate in and enjoys social situations.
- The individual has no behavior problems difficult to manage in the group setting, such as combativeness, severe agitation, wandering, or incontinence.
- The individual does not have concurrent medical or psychiatric conditions (including severe psychosis) that might put him or her or others in the group at risk.
- The individual understands the purpose of the support group, is interested, and freely gives consent to participate.
- The individual has a caregiver or someone who is willing to serve as a contact person for the group facilitator.

LEVEL AND ASSESSMENT
OF COGNITIVE FUNCTIONING

Individuals with only mild cognitive impairment will be best able to engage in and benefit from the support group. Cognitive functioning can be assessed through formal testing as well as informal responses to interview questions.

The Folstein Mini-Mental Status Exam (MMSE)[1] is one standardized tool that has been widely used to screen for cognitive impairment. Orientation, attention, recall, and language are among the areas covered. The MMSE requires only a brief time to administer, but training in properly conducting it is required. Any awkwardness a person may feel in introducing the test may be diffused by explaining honestly to the individual what the MMSE is for and that it is only one part of the routine screening process.

It is difficult to find consensus in the literature on the correlation between specific MMSE scores and levels of impairment. However, an initial score can be used as a baseline against which to compare future changes in functioning. This may be helpful when reevaluating the individuals for continued group participation.

For the support group model in this book, a score of 18 or above (out of a possible 30) was used as the cut-off point signifying mild cognitive impairment. However, this is only a suggested guideline because test scores alone may not give a complete or accurate representation of an individual's abilities, and the participants may also exhibit cognitive fluctuations on a daily basis. For this reason, it is important for the group facilitator to also ask the individual to discuss perceptions of and reactions to his or her confusion and memory loss. Impressions formed from this process can be supplemented by those of the caregivers or family members who are asked separately about the individual's cognitive, social, behavioral, and functional status. See Chapter 2 for sample interviews with the participants and their caregivers.

---

[1]Folstein, M.F., Folstein, S., & McHugh, P.R. (1975). Mini-mental state: A practical method for grading the cognitive state of patients for the clinician. *Journal of Psychiatric Research, 12,* 189–198.

OBTAINING AND
REVIEWING MEDICAL RECORDS

It is unfortunately still the case that many people are mis-diagnosed or simply misperceived as having Alzheimer's disease when in fact they do not. Because the purpose of this group model is to provide information and support about the illness to those who must truly cope with it, it is crucial that only people with Alzheimer's disease or other related disorders participate in the support group and that people with reversible causes of dementia (e.g., depression) not be included. One way of ensuring that everyone in the group belongs in the group is to have all diagnostic records reviewed by a qualified medical profes-sional. A form with the information requested in Figure 1 may be used to obtain the necessary consent.

Although a definite diagnosis of Alzheimer's disease can be made only upon autopsy, the disease can usually be identified if all other possible conditions that cause de-mentia are ruled out. In specialized settings that use standardized diagnostic criteria, clinical diagnosis of Alzheimer's disease now approaches 90% concordance with subsequent neuropathological diagnosis.[2] Thus, at the very least, it is important for the facilitator to find out from family members or a caregiver what type of "workup" had been done and who did it. Individuals who have not had a comprehensive diagnostic evaluation should be encouraged to do so before joining the group.

OTHER DEMENTIA-RELATED DIAGNOSES

There are other illnesses besides Alzheimer's disease that cause symptoms of dementia. A thorough evaluation is

---

[2]U.S. Department of Health and Human Services. (1994). *Seventh report of the Council on Alzheimer's Disease Progress in Research.* Washington, DC: Author.

22

required to determine whether the condition is treatable (e.g., depression), or progressive and irreversible (e.g., multi-infarct dementia).

Those with treatable, reversible symptoms obviously have different circumstances to deal with, and therefore would not be appropriate for this particular support group. In most cases of irreversible dementia, the ramifications of the symptoms are similar enough that participants may find common ground in the group even if their diagnoses vary. For example, a group participant who has dementia secondary to Parkinson's disease may have similar cognitive impairment to a participant with Alzheimer's disease, but have additional neurological difficulties, such as rigidity or tremors, that would need to be acknowledged.

If group members do have multiple dementia-related diagnoses, the facilitator is advised to become familiar with what is the same or different among their symptoms. The facilitator should keep in mind any distinctions about what is appropriate to generalize and clarify them during group discussions.

WILLINGNESS TO
ACKNOWLEDGE AND DISCUSS THE ILLNESS

Individuals are not routinely told by physicians, service providers, or family members that their diagnosis is Alzheimer's disease when it is determined. And individuals who are told the diagnosis do not always accept it or admit their difficulties. A group facilitator needs to carefully consider this when selecting group participants because the service is recommended only for those who are aware of and are seeking information about their condition.

Some people with Alzheimer's disease and/or their family members react to news of the diagnosis with staunch denial. This may be a necessary initial defense

CONSENT TO REQUEST INFORMATION

Patient's name: _____

Birthdate: _____

I hereby request that information be sent from my medical record in the office of:

Medical professional: _____

Address: _____

City, state, ZIP code: _____

Telephone: _____

To be sent for review to:

Agency name: _____

Address: _____

For the purpose of: Participation in a support group for individuals with early-stage Alzheimer's disease

The specific information requested is: Summary report of diagnostic evaluation of dementia

Patient's signature: _____

Date: _____

Guardian's or authorized representative's signature: _____

Date: _____

If signed by other than patient, indicate relationship:

Developing Support Groups for Individuals with Early-Stage
Alzheimer's Disease: Planning, Implementation, and Evaluation
by Robyn Yale   © 1995 Robyn Yale

Figure 1. A group leader will need a signed consent form before medical information can be released for review. This figure is an example of a request form that can be used.

against emotional pain, or it may be typical of a long-standing dysfunctional coping style. Each individual works through the difficult process of acceptance differently; some eventually move beyond denial, others remain steadfast in it, and many vacillate in and out of denial over a period of time. Furthermore, what may appear to be denial may in some instances be the individual actually forgetting about the diagnosis.

All too frequently, however, individuals are simply excluded from discussing their diagnosis because it is assumed that they will not understand or that they will have an unmanageable reaction. There is a tendency for professionals, as well as family members, to depersonalize the individual as a result of not only the symptoms but also their own discomfort with talking about the illness directly with the person who has it. In some cases, it is not realistic or appropriate to have such frank discussions, but even individuals with Alzheimer's disease who are capable of expressing their feelings and concerns are often denied this opportunity.

The issue of whether individuals should be told that their diagnosis is Alzheimer's disease is, then, a delicate and controversial one. There is little consensus on this issue, although it arises in many service settings (including diagnostic clinics, caregiver support groups, day programs, and information and referral centers). Each situation has a unique constellation of determining factors to examine, including whether the individual has asked for information, has a high level of insight and cognitive functioning, and has a family who has communicated openly during previous times of crisis or transition. Unfortunately, it is not usually within the role of one particular professional or agency to explore these circumstances with each person and family on a case-by-case basis. The result is often a lack of attention, guidance, and follow-up support at this crucial point in the disease course.

Figure 2 is a fact sheet developed by the Alzheimer's Association that offers guidelines for discussing with an individual his or her illness.

Careful thought about these issues is important, then, to clarify the procedures needed in selecting group participants. It may not matter as much that people acknowledge their illness if the format of the group has more recreation and less discussion. In the model discussed throughout this book, though, the topic of Alzheimer's disease is sure to arise in the group and should therefore be addressed at the time of intake screening. This also gives the facilitator a basis for later reviewing the purpose and ground rules of the group with its members.

CONCLUSION

Those who use denial to cope with Alzheimer's disease are less likely to seek out a support group focused on the illness, and this type of group is not right for everyone. There may also be diverse agendas or styles operating within one family system. For example, an adult daughter may want her father to participate in the group so that the facilitator will tell him that he has Alzheimer's disease. Of course, the facilitator's role is not to confront, advise, or debate the diagnosis but to make the support group available to those who are interested in and appropriate for it. This can best be determined by a structured selection process (see Chapter 2) in which each potential group member's perception and understanding of the illness are assessed. The guidelines also incorporate the other criteria recommended for choosing group participants that have been reviewed in this chapter.

FAMILY AND FRIENDS

When you learn that a member of your family has Alzheimer's disease, you may become overwhelmed by feelings of confusion, guilt and loneliness. Moreover, as you assume the role of caregiver, you may feel hesitant to reveal the diagnosis to the rest of the family, to friends, and—perhaps most importantly—to the person with the disease, for fear their reactions will be difficult to manage. Following are some guidelines that you may use to decide how to discuss the disease with others.

ACTION STEPS

Consider the person diagnosed.

■ In deciding whether or not to tell the person about the diagnosis, respect his/her right to know what's wrong, but also be sensitive to the person's feelings and emotional state, medical condition, and ability to remember, reason and make decisions.

■ Keep in mind that the person with Alzheimer's may suspect that something is wrong long before a doctor reaches a diagnosis. If you fail to give her any explanation, she may assume the worst. On the other hand, if you discuss the problem with her, she may feel relieved to learn that she has a physical illness, rather than a psychological one.

■ When you sense the time is right, provide the person with follow-up information you feel she would benefit from knowing, such as an explanation of symptoms and the importance of continued care. For example, you may say, "Mom, because of your memory and other problems, you may have to let people help you more than you have in the past." (Note: You don't have to use the phrase Alzheimer's disease if you think it might upset the person.)

■ Treat the person as an adult, and don't downplay the disease. As the disease progresses, remain open to the person's need to talk about his illness. The person may ask you about such activities as working, driving, or managing finances. Or the person may want to express such feelings as anger, frustration, and disappointment. Be aware of nonverbal signs of sadness, anger or anxiety, and respond with love and reassurance.

Inform family and friends.

■ Be honest about the person's condition. You'll probably feel relieved after discussing the disease with other family members and close friends. Be sure to explain that Alzheimer's is a medical condition and not a psychological or emotional disorder or contagious virus.

■ Provide others with adequate information on Alzheimer's disease, including a description of common symptoms. The more family and friends learn about the

TELLING THE PATIENT,

Furthermore, the informed person may be able to participate in important medical, legal, financial and personal planning, depending on the progression of the disease symptoms.

■ Rely on professional experience. You may want to inform the person about the diagnosis through a "family conference" with the patient, other caregivers and a social worker. You may also want to involve a physician who has experience working with cognitively impaired individuals.

■ Be sensitive to the person's reaction. He may not be able to understand all that the diagnosis means, or he may deny your explanation. If this is the case, it's probably best to accept his reaction and avoid further detailed explanations of the disease.

■ Reassure the person. Let the person know that you'll provide ongoing help and support, and do all you can to make your lives together fulfilling.

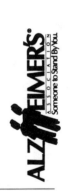

disease, the more comfortable they may feel around the person. Share educational material from the Alzheimer's Association, such as the brochure "When the Diagnosis is Alzheimer's." You may also want to invite close friends and family members to accompany you to a support group meeting sponsored by a local Chapter of the Alzheimer's Association.

■ Don't leave yourself out of the conversation. Explain how the responsibility of caregiving has affected your life or may change your life in the future, so that others will have a better sense of how they can help.

■ Ask for family support. Have several tasks in mind for people who say, "Please let me know if there's anything I can do to help you." Involving others in caregiving will help them better understand your situation and why you've made certain decisions.

■ Ask people to come for short visits, but suggest they call you before stopping. Keep in mind that the person may become anxious if too many people visit at one time. In addition, recommend specific activities such as playing a simple game, taking a walk, or looking through a book of photographs with the person.

(continued)

Figure 2. An important issue for families involves the decision to tell an individual if he or she has Alzheimer's disease. The Alzheimer's Association developed a fact sheet on this issue. (Reprinted with permission from the National Alzheimer's Association.)

Figure 2. *(continued)*

■ Don't overlook the role of children and teenagers in the life of your family member. Young children often are able to relate to a person who has limited verbal ability. Teenagers and young adults feel valued if they're offered an opportunity to spend time with the person or share some of your responsibilities.

■ Inform neighbors about the person's condition. Even if you've never socialized with your neighbors, they'll appreciate knowing the truth about the person's condition. They may have already observed the family member wandering through the neighborhood or acting strangely. If they understand the diagnosis, they'll be more likely to call if they sense the person needs help. Or they may volunteer to help you in an emergency.

Be true to yourself and to the person with Alzheimer's.

■ Realize that some friends and even family may drift out of your life. Some people may feel uncomfortable around the impaired person while others may not want to get involved in caregiving. Don't let these attitudes interfere with your commitment to caring for your family member and for yourself.

Donna Cohen, Ph.D., and Carl Eisdorfer, Ph.D., M.D. THE LOSS OF SELF: A FAMILY RESOURCE FOR THE CARE OF ALZHEIMER'S DISEASE AND RELATED DISORDERS. New York: New American Library, 1986.

"WHEN THE DIAGNOSIS IS ALZHEIMER'S." Alzheimer's Association, 1990.*

"IF YOU HAVE ALZHEIMER'S DISEASE: WHAT YOU SHOULD KNOW, WHAT YOU CAN DO." Alzheimer's Association, 1991.*

"ALZHEIMER'S DISEASE: ESPECIALLY FOR TEENAGERS." Alzheimer's Association, 1987.*

These materials are available through your local Chapter of the Alzheimer's Association, or the National office.

Notes

30

RESOURCES

One of the best places to turn for additional help is the Alzheimer's Association. The Alzheimer's Association has more than 200 Chapters and 1,600 support groups nationwide, where family members of people with Alzheimer's disease or a related disorder share their experiences, provide each other with emotional support, hear practical suggestions and learn to rebuild their lives. To locate a Chapter near you, call our toll-free number, listed below.

The primary resource for this fact sheet was Mary Barringer, RN.C., Partner, Professional Care Management Services, Springfield, Illinois.

Special thanks to the following Chapters of the Alzheimer's Association:

Dallas
Eastern Massachusetts
Honolulu
Northern Virginia
Puget Sound
St. Louis
Western North Carolina

ALZHEIMER'S ASSOCIATION
919 North Michigan Avenue
Chicago, IL 60611-1676
312-335-8700

1-800-272-3900
TDD: 312-335-8882

31

2

RECRUITING AND SELECTING GROUP PARTICIPANTS

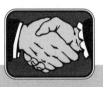

- Interviewing potential group participants
- The two-step participant selection process
- Handling denial during the selection process
- Individuals without caregivers
- Relevant background information
- Sample intake screening and interview forms
- The ongoing nature of participant assessment

The process and format used to select group participants should be just as systematic as the criteria set for this purpose. It is important for the facilitator to allow plenty of time for meeting potential group members and asking the questions that will help determine each individual's appropriateness for the program. Simultaneously, the facilitator can begin to learn about the backgrounds of those who will be enrolled and develop relationships with them. This chapter suggests methods and provides forms for use at this step.

INTERVIEWING
POTENTIAL GROUP PARTICIPANTS

Once the group facilitator has identified the ideal characteristics for group participants to have, he or she can begin to seek them out. A two-step process involving *both* the potential participants and their families in telephone and in-person interviewing is recommended. Although this is very time intensive, such thorough initial screening increases the chances that all who are ultimately selected for the group will have a successful experience.

THE TWO-STEP
PARTICIPANT SELECTION PROCESS

The selection process involves telephone intake screening followed by in-person interviewing. These interactions allow the facilitator to formally assess each person's appropriateness for the group as well as become acquainted more informally with group members and their families.

Time and care spent in lengthy telephone screening will reduce the incidence of unnecessary home or office visits so that only those who meet the selection criteria are interviewed. Multiple telephone calls to the same household may even be necessary if family members ask for time to think about the group and discuss it with the individual who might participate. Caregivers who have not yet fully faced the person's illness are one example of those who hesitate—and this in turn may depend on such factors as the recency of diagnosis and the severity of symptoms.

The facilitator can do the bulk of initial screening with a family member or caregiver, but it is advisable to also talk with the potential participant on the telephone to see how he or she responds to the idea of the group. If the reaction is resistance or confusion, it may indicate that the person is not right for the group. If instead there is interest and agreement, an interview appointment can then be made with the caregiver's assistance.

The in-person interview begins with an introduction given to the potential participant and caregiver together, and then each is interviewed separately. This can be expedited if two staff people are available—one to assess the individual's insight and behavior and one to seek the caregiver's perceptions of the individual's functioning and how he or she would do in a group.

The individual can be reassured that not everyone with memory loss experiences all of the things he or she will be asked about in the interview and that there are no "right" answers. Rather, a picture is painted of the person's experience, and the types of issues that will be discussed in the support group are simultaneously illustrated.

Figure 1 summarizes the basic questions the facilitator should ask the caregiver and potential participant during the initial telephone screening and in-person interviews. Complete sample interview forms appear later in this chapter.

HANDLING DENIAL
DURING THE SELECTION PROCESS

Even with well-defined selection criteria, the dynamics of interview situations are not always clear-cut. For example, people may acknowledge that they have memory loss during initial telephone contact but then deny this when the facilitator meets them in person. Or, they may be consistent throughout the interviewing but then be in denial during a group session. Such fluctuations are not uncommon and it is wise to anticipate them.

However, there are likely to be many individuals who will welcome the opportunity to discuss the illness with the facilitator because they have long felt isolated and misunderstood. Even those who are guarded at first may open up in the course of an interview. Rapport can be built by choosing tactful (but not evasive) language, such as "changes that occur as one gets older," or using the term "memory loss" rather than Alzheimer's disease. In the research discussed in Chapter 9, several of the individuals enjoyed the attention and empathy from the interview situation so much that they disclosed even more than they were asked to after it was concluded. In addition, some who at first did not say what their diagnosis was listened with interest when the group was described and then admitted their own difficulties.

Making the most of the interview with each potential group member takes patience and perhaps ingenuity. A good rule of thumb is for the facilitator to "back off" im-

SCREENING AND INTERVIEWING
POTENTIAL SUPPORT GROUP PARTICIPANTS

Initial Telephone Screening

QUESTIONS TO ASK THE CAREGIVER:

1. **Individual's history**
   - Does the individual have a documented diagnosis of Alzheimer's disease or other dementia?
   - How was the diagnosis determined, and by whom?
   - When were symptoms of dementia noticed? When was it diagnosed?
   - Are there any other significant medical or psychiatric conditions?

2. **Individual's awareness of diagnosis**
   - What was the person told about his or her condition? When and by whom?
   - What was his or her reaction?

- To what extent does the individual discuss the illness, and what does he or she typically say about it?

- To what extent do the individual and his or her family discuss the illness together?

- Has the individual sought information and support about the illness? If yes, in what ways?

3. **Individual's suitability for group participation**

- Is the individual able to verbally communicate his or her thoughts and feelings about the illness?

- Are there any speech or comprehension difficulties?

- Do you think the individual would be able to stay interested and focused on a group for 1–1½ hours?

- Does the individual have any behavior problems, such as agitation?

(continued)

Developing Support Groups for Individuals with Early-Stage Alzheimer's Disease: Planning, Implementation, and Evaluation by Robyn Yale   © 1995 Robyn Yale

Figure 1.   Questions a facilitator should ask the caregiver and potential participant during the initial telephone screening and in-person interview.

Figure 1. *(continued)*

- Are there any other problems that might be difficult to manage in this group setting, such as incontinence, wandering, and so forth?

- How does the individual do in social situations?

4. **Caregiver involvement**

- Is there a caregiver who will maintain contact with the facilitator?

- What is the caregiver's relationship and involvement with the individual?

- How much does the caregiver seem to understand and accept about the person's diagnosis?

- Does the caregiver want the individual to be in this support group?

5. **Meeting logistics**

- How will the individual be transported to and from meetings?

- Will the individual be escorted and supervised before and after meetings?

- Does the individual have any mobility problems?

- Are the planned times and location of meetings convenient?

QUESTIONS TO ASK THE POTENTIAL PARTICIPANT:

1. Interest in group

- Are you interested in attending a discussion and/or support group focused on understanding and coping with memory problems?

2. Consent to be interviewed

- Is it okay with you if I set up a time to meet with you and a family member to talk about this further?

In-Person Interviewing

QUESTIONS TO ASK THE CAREGIVER:

1. The individual's status

- How is the individual functioning in terms of self-care, cognition, behavior, and so forth?

(continued)

Figure 1. *(continued)*

- Are there impairments about which the individual is particularly concerned?

- Does the individual seem excessively depressed, worried, or anxious?

2. **The reaction of the individual with Alzheimer's disease to the illness**

- How has the person's life changed as a result of Alzheimer's disease?

- How has the person adjusted to these changes (in terms of lifestyle, emotional reaction, etc.)?

- How does the person currently spend his or her time (in terms of any paid or volunteer work, leisure activities or interests, social and family life, etc.)?

3. **The caregiver's reaction to the individual's illness**

- What about the illness is most difficult for the caregiver?

- How is the caregiver feeling and managing?

- Is the caregiver aware of and/or using any support services?

QUESTIONS TO ASK THE POTENTIAL PARTICIPANT:

1. Perception of memory problem

- Are you having any problems with memory and/or daily functioning?

- What do you think is causing these problems?

- What have you been told about the possible cause, and by whom?

- Have you sought any further information? From whom and where?

2. Lifestyle

- Has your life changed at all since these problems began?

- How do you feel about the changes in your life?

- How do you spend your time, in terms of work, social life, hobbies, and activities?

3. Cognitive testing

- May I do a brief test of your memory today?

(continued)

Figure 1. *(continued)*

- As a general guideline, if the potential participant scores above 18 on the Folstein Mini-Mental Status Exam (MMSE), he or she will be at an appropriate level of cognitive functioning for the support group. However, impressions from the rest of the assessment interview must also be considered so that this cutoff point is not the sole basis for selecting group participants.

4. **Group participation**

- Have you ever been in a support or discussion group?

- Would you like to be in this group with others who will be learning and talking about coping with memory problems?

mediately from people who deny their illness. The best procedure in these cases is to politely thank them for their time and conclude the conversation. However, with someone who is open to discussing the illness, the facilitator can be very direct in introducing the focus of the group and asking whether he or she would like to participate.

INDIVIDUALS WITHOUT CAREGIVERS

It is ideal if each group participant has a caregiver who can provide background information, transportation to meetings, and liaison with the group facilitator. This may or may not be a family member or someone who lives with the individual, but should be someone with whom there is familiarity and frequent contact.

However, many people with Alzheimer's disease (particularly in the early stages) do not have caregivers. Some live alone and some have relatives out of the region. It would be unfortunate if a person who was otherwise perfect for the group were denied the opportunity to participate just for this reason. If possible, the facilitator might seek the services of a case manager or other professional who could monitor the participant and provide other supportive services.

There may also be instances where an individual has a caregiver who cannot or will not be involved as a contact person. Most often, though, caregivers who seek out the support group for their relatives are appreciative and glad to offer any assistance needed by the facilitator.

RELEVANT BACKGROUND INFORMATION

Background information provides important history about each individual as well as about his or her unique experience with the illness. Learning as much as possible about participants catalyzes the building of relationships, which are the foundation of the group process.

The format of the group will help to determine which areas of questioning should be emphasized. For example, if the facilitator is offering a concurrent support group for family members, he or she may want to assess in detail how they are coping with the stress of caregiving. The focus will also be different if, for instance, the program has a recreational or vocational component and in-depth information about relevant skills and interests is needed. In other cases, if the facilitator is doing research in conjunction with the support group, he or she is likely to need formal assessment tools to measure the areas of exploration.

SAMPLE INTAKE
SCREENING AND INTERVIEW FORMS

Figures 2, 3, and 4 are provided as sample intake screening and interview forms. The telephone intake screening allows the facilitator to identify potential group participants who meet the selection criteria as well as to collect some demographic information. The in-person interviews introduce the facilitator to the potential participants and their caregivers and further solidify his or her impressions of each person's appropriateness for the group.

These particular forms are not intended for collecting research, diagnostic, or other unrelated data. If the facilitator wants to document certain characteristics or trends or if the group focus requires different areas of assessment, he or she may adapt these forms for individualized practice settings or aims.

THE ONGOING NATURE
OF PARTICIPANT ASSESSMENT

Selecting group participants is based only in part on how they respond to the interviews. The other element is intuition, which of course cannot be foolproof. Errors may become apparent as the group begins or as a participant who was assessed at one level begins to experience a decline in functioning. For these reasons, it is advisable to explain during initial interviewing that evaluation of appropriateness for the group will be ongoing. That is, if the facilitator becomes concerned about how someone is doing, the plan will be to discuss it with the individual and his or her family, and *decide together* whether he or she should continue in the group. A more formal reassessment can occur periodically if a break is planned after a time-limited session (e.g., an 8-week group will be followed by 2 weeks off before it begins again). At this time, the group leader can modify or administer the same interview and also ask group participants to evaluate the sessions.

CONCLUSION

Selection of support group participants should be based on a careful assessment process. Interviews with potential participants and their caregivers (when available) should be conducted first on the telephone and then in person. This allows for a thorough exploration of suitability for and interest in the group while also providing important background information about each individual. The sample questionnaires in this chapter may be used initially as well as for the reevaluation of group participants over time.

TELEPHONE INTAKE/SCREENING

Date: ___/___/___ Staff person: _____ Potential participant: _____

1. Contact person is a: Potential participant: _____ Caregiver: _____
   Professional: _____ Other (specify): _____

2. Relationship to potential participant: Self: _____ Relative (specify): _____
   Professional (e.g., case worker, therapist): _____
   Other (specify): _____

3. Contact person's name, address, and telephone number:
   _____
   _____
   _____

4. If different, list ongoing contact person's name, address, and telephone number:
   _____
   _____
   _____

   Relationship to participant: _____

5. Referred to group by: Family: _____   Friend: _____

    Agency or professional   (Name: _____   Telephone: _____

    Media or other publicity (specify): _____

    Other: _____

INFORMATION ABOUT THE INDIVIDUAL WITH ALZHEIMER'S DISEASE:

Name: _____

Address: _____

Telephone: _____

6. When were symptoms of confusion and/or memory loss first noticed? ____ / ____ (month/year)

_____

(continued)

Developing Support Groups for Individuals with Early-Stage
Alzheimer's Disease: Planning, Implementation, and Evaluation
by Robyn Yale   © 1995 Robyn Yale

Figure 2. A questionnaire form used to record vital information during the initial telephone screening process. This form is not intended to collect research, diagnostic, or other unrelated data. It is used as the first step in determining if an individual might be appropriate for group support.

49

Figure 2. *(continued)*

7. When were these symptoms first evaluated? _____ / _____ (month/year)

8. When were symptoms most recently evaluated? _____ / _____ (month/year)

9. What was the diagnosis(es)? _____

_____

10. Who determined this diagnosis? Name: _____

Telephone: _____

11. List the individual's primary physician, if different:

Name: _____

Address: _____

_____

Telephone: _____

12. Was the individual informed of his or her diagnosis? Yes: _____ No: _____

13. Who informed the individual of the diagnosis?

Physician or other clinicians: _____

Family (specify): _____

Other (specify): _____

Comments:

14. When was the individual informed of his or her diagnosis? ____/____ (month/year)

15. What was the individual told about his or her diagnosis? _____

_____

_____

16. Does the individual discuss his or her illness much?   Yes: ____   No: ____

17. What kinds of things does he or she say about it? _____

_____

_____

_____

(continued)

51

Figure 2. *(continued)*

18. Is the individual able to clearly communicate his or her thoughts? Yes: _____ No: _____

19. Are there any speech or comprehension problems? Yes: _____ No: _____

   Describe:

20. Can the individual tell you how he or she feels? Yes: _____ No: _____

   Comments:

21. Does the individual generally do well in social situations? Yes: _____ No: _____

   Comments:

22. What social activities is the individual currently involved in? _____

23. Does the individual have any other major medical diagnoses? Yes: _____ No: _____

   List:

24. Has the individual had any problems for which he or she has seen a psychiatrist? Yes: _____ No: _____

    List:

25. Is the individual currently in therapy? Yes: _____ No: _____ If yes, please specify type:

    Individual: _____

    Family: _____

    Group: _____

    Other: _____

    Name of clinician: _____

26. Is the individual currently taking any medications? Yes: _____ No: _____

    List all medications:

27. In your opinion, does the individual abuse alcohol or medications? Yes: _____ No: _____

    Explain:

    _____

(continued)

53

Figure 2. *(continued)*

28. Do you have any current concerns about the individual's mood? If yes, please specify:

   Anxiety: _____ Depression: _____ Delusions: _____ Other (specify): _____ None: _____

   Comments:

29. Are there any current behavior problems? If yes, please specify:

   Combativeness: _____ Wandering: _____ Agitation: _____ Other (specify): _____
   None: _____

   Comments:

30. Could the individual sit through a 1½-hour session without bowel or bladder accidents? Yes: _____ No: _____

31. Do you think the individual could sit in a 1½-hour group session and remain interested? Yes: _____ No: _____

32. Do you think the individual can understand our explanation of the group and sign consent to participate?
   Yes: _____ No: _____

33. Is the individual ambulatory?

   Ambulates independently: _____ Ambulates with the assistance of another person: _____

   Ambulates with assistive device: _____ Needs a wheelchair: _____

34. How will the individual get to the group sessions? _____

_____

35. What is the individual's age? _____

36. What is the individual's gender?   Male: _____   Female: _____

37. What is the individual's education level?

Less than high school: _____   High school graduate: _____   Some college: _____

College graduate: _____   Postgraduate or professional: _____

38. What is the individual's race or ethnic background?

Native American: _____   Asian: _____   African American: _____   Hispanic: _____

Caucasian: _____   Other (specify): _____

39. Where is the individual's place of birth? _____

40. Is the individual's primary language English?   Yes: _____   No: _____

_____

(continued)

55

Figure 2. *(continued)*

41. What is the individual's living arrangement?

    Home (alone): _____ Home (with spouse and/or other relatives): _____

    Home (with nonrelatives): _____ Residential care facility: _____ Other (specify): _____

    Comments:

INFORMATION ABOUT THE CAREGIVER:

1. Is the caregiver willing to be interviewed and be an ongoing contact person? Yes: _____ No: _____

2. Did the caregiver know the individual before the memory problem began? Yes: _____ No: _____

    Length of relationship: _____

3. How often does the caregiver have contact with the individual?

    Daily: _____

    Several times a week: _____

    Weekly: _____

    Several times a month: _____

    Monthly: _____

Type of contact:

4. What is the caregiver's age? ____

5. What is the caregiver's gender?   Male: ____   Female: ____

6. What is the caregiver's race or ethnic background?

   Native American: ____   Asian: ____   African American: ____

   Hispanic: ____   Caucasian: ____   Other (specify): ____

7. Is the caregiver's primary language English?   Yes: ____   No: ____

8. Is the caregiver employed? Please mark the answer that best applies.

   Full time: ____   Part time: ____   Not employed: ____

9. How does the caregiver rate his or her own health status?

   Excellent: ____   Good: ____   Fair: ____   Poor: ____

(continued)

Figure 2. *(continued)*

DETERMINING WHETHER TO CONDUCT AN IN-PERSON INTERVIEW:

To Be Completed by the Facilitator After the Telephone Interview

1. What was the potential participant's response (on the telephone) to the idea of being in a group?

2. Did he or she agree (on the telephone) to meet for an interview?   Yes: _____   No: _____

3. If the individual does not meet screening criteria, note reason: _____

   _____
   _____

4. If the individual does meet screening criteria but cannot otherwise participate in the group, note reason:

   _____
   _____
   _____

5. Preference for group location: _____

6. Preference for a group meeting time: _____

7. Interview appointment:

    Date: _____

    Time: _____

    Place: _____

8. Special notes:

59

INTERVIEWING THE INDIVIDUAL WITH ALZHEIMER'S DISEASE

Date: _____ / _____ / _____   Staff person: _____   Individual's name: _____

1. What, if any, problems are you having with confusion or memory loss?

2. Please tell me if you have any problems with confusing the:
   a. Times of the day or days
   b. People
   c. Places you find yourself
   d. None of the above
   Comments:

3. Do you have difficulty with things like:
   a. Finding the right words or recalling words or names
   b. Reading or recalling some things you read
   c. Managing your personal or household finances
   d. Driving
   e. None of the above
   Comments:

4. Are there any other areas we have not discussed that are troublesome for you?

5. What do you think is the cause of these difficulties you have been experiencing?

6. Have you been told anything by a doctor or anyone else about the cause or diagnosis of these problems? If so, what?

7. Have you tried to get more information about your condition, for example, from medical professionals, agencies, family members, or books?

_____

(continued)

Developing Support Groups for Individuals with Early-Stage Alzheimer's Disease: Planning, Implementation, and Evaluation by Robyn Yale   © 1995 Robyn Yale

Figure 3. A questionnaire form used to record information discussed between the individual with early-stage Alzheimer's disease and the group facilitator during the in-person interview. A facilitator may adapt this form in order to work with his or her own goals for a support group.

61

Figure 3. *(continued)*

8. Is there any particular information about your illness you would like to get?

9. Do you usually talk to anyone about your illness or the problems you have been experiencing? If so, who?

10. Is there anyone else you would like to talk to about the problems you have been experiencing? If so, who?

11. Think back to before these problems began. How has your life changed since you first noticed that you had a problem? How do you feel about this?

12. I would like to ask about how you spend your time now. Are you doing any paid or volunteer work?

13. Were you previously involved in paid or volunteer work?

14. What types of hobbies, interests, and leisure activities are you doing now?

15. Are there any hobbies or activities you did in the past that you are not doing anymore?

16. Tell me about your social life. Do you:
    a. Belong to clubs
    b. Go to church or other religious functions
    c. See friends regularly
    d. Other (specify):

    Comments:

(continued)

Figure 3. *(continued)*

17. Who are the people closest to you?

    a. Spouse

    b. Children

    c. Other relatives (specify):

    d. Friends

    e. Other (specify):

18. Have your relationships with the people identified above changed in any way? Please explain.

19. How would you say you have been feeling in general?

20. How would you say that your mood has been over the past month (e.g., cheerful, sad, irritable)?

21. Do you worry much? If so, what kinds of things do you worry about?

22. I am here today to invite you to join a support group for people who are having problems similar to yours. Have you ever been in a support group or discussion group before? If yes, how did you like it?

23. Now I need to do some short testing of your memory and then we'll be finished.

[At this point the Folstein Mini-Mental Status Exam (MMSE) should be administered.]
MMSE score: _____

Thank you for your patience and cooperation!

Staff Observations/Notes (insight, communication, orientation, family interaction, etc.):

INTERVIEWING THE CAREGIVER

Date: ___ / ___ / ___   Staff person: _____   Caregiver's name: _____

1. With what kinds of things do you regularly need to assist the individual who has Alzheimer's disease (e.g., self-care, other activities of daily living)?

2. Are there any specific problematic behaviors (e.g., the individual repeating questions or following you around) with which you must deal?

3. Can you give some examples of the individual's cognitive difficulties (e.g., word finding, understanding things you explain)?

4. Does the individual ever talk with you about the problems he or she has been having? If so, what does he or she say?

5. What does the individual think is the cause of these problems?

6. What was the individual told about the diagnosis of these problems and by whom?

7. Does the individual talk to anyone else about the diagnosis or the problems he or she has been having? If so, who?

8. Has the individual tried to get more information about the problems he or she has been having? If so, from where?

(continued)

Developing Support Groups for Individuals with Early-Stage Alzheimer's Disease: Planning, Implementation, and Evaluation by Robyn Yale © 1995 Robyn Yale

Figure 4. A questionnaire form used to record information discussed between the caregiver and the group facilitator during the in-person interview.

Figure 4. *(continued)*

9. Think back to before these problems began. How has the individual's life changed since the time these problems began? How do you think he or she feels about this?

10. Is the individual currently doing any paid or volunteer work?

11. How is this a change from the individual's previous work life?

    a. Change in responsibilities

    b. Works fewer hours

    c. Stopped working

    d. Started new type of work

    e. Other (specify):

12. What types of hobbies, interests, and leisure activities does the individual do now?

13. Are there any hobbies or activities he or she did in the past that he or she does not do anymore?

14. Tell me about the individual's social life. Does he or she:

    a. Belong to clubs
    b. Go to church or other religious functions
    c. See friends regularly
    d. Other (specify):

    Comments:

(continued)

Figure 4. *(continued)*

15. Are there ways in which the individual's social life has changed since the onset of the illness?

16. Who are the people closest to the individual?

    a. Spouse

    b. Children

    c. Other relatives (specify):

    d. Friends

    e. Other (specify):

17. Is there any way in which the individual's relationships with the people identified above have changed?

18. Are there ways in which things at home have changed (e.g., he or she used to manage finances but can no longer do so)?

19. Has the individual completed a:

a. Power of attorney for health care

b. Power of attorney for finances

c. Both of the above

d. Neither of the above

20. Are there any changes we have not discussed that are troublesome for the individual?

21. How would you say the individual's mood has been in the past month?

22. Do his or her moods change frequently or extremely? If yes, please describe.

23. Does the individual worry much? If so, about what kinds of things?

71

(continued)

Figure 4. *(continued)*

24. Are there any changes we have not discussed that are troublesome for you as a caregiver?

25. In general, how would you say you are managing with the caregiving responsibilities?

26. Do you have concerns about your own mood or stress level?

27. Have you yourself sought more information about the individual's illness? If so, from where?

28. Have you used any community services, such as caregiver support groups, day or in-home respite care, counseling, and so forth?

29. Would you like information on these or other services?

30. I am here today to invite the individual to join a support group for people who are having problems similar to his or her own. Has he or she ever been in a support or discussion group before? If so, how did it work out?

31. Where will you be during the group sessions?

32. List name, address, and telephone number of person(s) to contact in case of an emergency:

Thank you for your patience and cooperation!

Staff Observation/Notes: (caregiver's view of symptoms, caregiver functioning, family interaction, etc.):

3

SELECTING AND WORKING WITH GROUP FACILITATORS

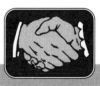

- Recommended facilitator qualifications
- Specialized training for support group leaders
- Supervision and consultation with facilitators
- Volunteer versus paid facilitators
- Cofacilitators or other supplemental personnel

The highly specialized nature of support groups for individuals with early-stage Alzheimer's disease requires that such groups be led by facilitators with solid credentials and experience. Initial orientation and training, along with ongoing monitoring of group leaders, increase the likelihood that facilitators will have the skills to do well in this challenging role. This chapter covers important aspects of choosing, preparing, and overseeing facilitators for leading this particular type of support group.

RECOMMENDED FACILITATOR QUALIFICATIONS

A good group leader must be able to establish a relationship with each of the members. This very basic, yet important, element of group facilitation also begets the building of rapport and trust among participants so that they develop a sense of comfort and safety, as well as camaraderie with one another.

Personal qualities that make individuals successful support group facilitators include empathy, patience, and good communication skills. Although many self-help groups (including those for the caregivers of people with Alzheimer's disease) are led by laypersons with relevant life experience, there is a general concern and consensus that groups for individuals with dementia require a different level of leadership skill.

The qualifications recommended for facilitators of these groups, then, include the following:

1. Because of the sensitive nature of issues likely to arise in the group, facilitators should ideally have a background in mental health and be licensed thera-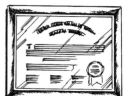pists. However, in some situations or regions there may not be anyone with these credentials available. Nonlicensed professionals or even other trained personnel who meet the other qualifications below may be considered to conduct groups, but are advised to seek appropriate professional supervision (e.g., from a licensed clinical social worker; marriage, family, and child counselor; psychologist; psychiatrist).

2. Formal training and/or previous experience in group work are also important. In addition to the facilitation skills required in any group setting, unique dynamics require specific interventions in the group process because of each participant's cognitive impairment.

3. Group facilitators should have a solid background in dementia, including direct experience working with people with Alzheimer's disease as well as their families. An overview of the illness, knowledge of communication and behavior management techniques, familiarity with the resources in the community, and a good grasp of the psychosocial and care-planning issues are all likely to be called upon in group discussions.

4. Other qualifications that are tailored to a specific program format may be important. For example, if there will be a recreational component or an educational fo-

cus, the facilitator should be skilled and experienced in providing these services to individuals with dementia.

SPECIALIZED TRAINING FOR SUPPORT GROUP LEADERS

Once qualified facilitators have been identified, standardized orientation and training should be provided to ensure that the support groups are conducted with a consistent and constructive approach. The following are recommended areas that should be included in this orientation and training:

- A basic orientation to the issues and abilities specific to people with early-stage Alzheimer's disease and their families
- The protocol established for setting up groups, including interviewing potential participants and administering any assessment tools (e.g., the Folstein Mini-Mental Status Exam)
- An overview of the topics, dynamics, and facilitation techniques unique to group work with people who have cognitive impairment
- Attention to any special focus or subpopulation the group might have (e.g., issues of cultural diversity, the different needs of younger individuals with dementia)
- Administrative procedures (e.g., dealing with emergencies, attending to changes in the individuals' status, communication with participants' family members)
- Role plays (i.e., to allow facilitators to experience simulated group characters and interactions) (see Chapter 8)

The orientation and training need to be provided by individuals with experience in conducting support groups for individuals with early-stage Alzheimer's disease as well as in training facilitators. Didactic presentation of material can be combined with opportunities to observe and gradually assume supervised responsibility for leading the group.

Training workshops allow more potential facilitators to receive orientation and administrative guidelines at the same time and to discuss and practice group leadership skills. Role plays are an effective tool for enacting hypothetical group sessions. Trainees can then anticipate the situations and people they may actually encounter and talk about strategies, feelings, and concerns that arise as they react to them. The role plays in Chapter 8 incorporate some of the personality types found in most typical group settings as well as some that are unique to the support groups for people with early-stage Alzheimer's disease.

Trainees can also sit in on the process of interviewing and selecting actual group participants. Role plays may also be useful in this situation to supplement preparation for the delicate art of talking one-to-one with individuals about their diagnosis of Alzheimer's disease. Trainees can also observe or cofacilitate actual sessions with an experienced leader before attempting to do them alone.

The amount of time needed for this orientation and training period is likely to be different for each facilitator depending on his or her background, learning style, and level of comfort with starting a support group. Therefore, if possible, there should be flexibility in adapting the amount, level, and format of training to each individual's previous experience.

SUPERVISION AND CONSULTATION WITH FACILITATORS

Group facilitators should have ongoing supervision and/or consultation available as follow-up to the initial orientation and training. This may be provided by qualified staff from the agency sponsoring the support group, by colleagues in peer groups, or by a licensed professional who is privately retained. Such outside expertise will be invaluable in assisting new facilitators to problem-solve, debrief, plan, refine skills, and deal with any of their own feelings and issues that may be aroused by their work in the group.

VOLUNTEER VERSUS PAID FACILITATORS

Although many self-help groups are facilitated by laypersons who volunteer their time, the consensus in the dementia field seems to be that support groups for individuals with Alzheimer's disease should be conducted by professionals. It is likely to be difficult to find professionals willing to provide this service without being paid for their time. Furthermore, the facilitator's commitment is substantial because training is involved, selecting participants is quite time consuming, and time is required not only for leading the group but also for preparatory and follow-up work. Compensation may be offered to facilitators by the agency sponsoring the group for all, some, or none of these related activities.

COFACILITATORS OR OTHER SUPPLEMENTAL PERSONNEL

There are many advantages to having more than one person involved in running group sessions. If a facilitator chooses to have additional people, he or she must clearly delineate the role of each person and be aware that there are many possible configurations.

Supplemental personnel may act as cofacilitators in group discussion or other activity (e.g., recreation, education). In this format, cofacilitators can either equally share responsibility for the group focus, or they can divide their attention so that one sustains the program while the other assists and responds to any extraneous needs of members (e.g., to have a stretch).

Another possible format is to have one facilitator in the group and a second person who has other outside tasks. For instance, recruiting and enrolling participants, observing and evaluating group sessions, welcoming and orienting members when they arrive at meetings, reassuring and assisting families, and managing disruptive behaviors or other unanticipated events are all ways in which additional personnel can be very useful.

The decision to have supplemental personnel may be affected by the amount of funding available. If cofacilitators are expected to assume joint and equal responsibilities, they will need to have similar credentials and capabilities and undergo the training described above. In this case, they would each have to be compensated similarly for their services. However, if supplemental personnel commit less time or have less significant responsibilities (or if they are trainees), different compensation may be negotiated and arranged.

Decisions about the number of personnel involved with the group may also depend on the size of the group. A larger group (e.g., eight members) is likely to have more need for and more comfort with a second staff person than a small group might (e.g., four members).

Whether or not more than one person is staffing a group, the facilitator might consider identifying someone in his or her agency or community who has the appropriate expertise to act as a back-up person. It helps to know there is someone the facilitator can count on in the event of an emergency or if the group facilitator is unable to attend a session.

CONCLUSION

The success of a support group for individuals with early-stage Alzheimer's disease depends greatly on the person who facilitates it. For this reason, it is important to carefully select facilitators with a relevant background, equip them with additional knowledge and skills, and provide ongoing supervision. Compensation for facilitators and the roles of any additional personnel will need to be clearly specified.

4

Setting Up a Support Group

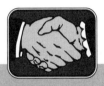

- Support group structure
- Open-ended versus time-limited groups
- Duration of group sessions
- Assessing and handling changes in participants' appropriateness for the group
- Open versus closed enrollment
- Meeting attendance, frequency, and length
- Time and place of meetings
- Group size
- Composition of the membership
- Accommodating cultural diversity

There are many logistical questions to be resolved before a support group can be formed. For example, the structure and duration of meetings, as well as the composition of the membership, are factors that may vary from one group setting to another. This chapter explores options and makes recommendations for this point in the planning process.

SUPPORT GROUP STRUCTURE

Services for individuals with early-stage dementia are still relatively new and have not yet been standardized. Thus, various types of innovative programs have reported success although they have differences in features. Because there are no formalized guidelines, there are no "right" decisions to be made about the structure and logistics of support group meetings. This chapter discusses the multiple options, considerations, and choices a facilitator or agency offering a group should think about and incorporate in the planning process.

OPEN-ENDED VERSUS TIME-LIMITED GROUPS

Groups may be set up to run on an ongoing basis or to have a finite number of sessions. This may depend in part on what resources are available to manage and sustain the program. It also requires clarifying whether the objective is to serve as many different clients as possible or to provide the same clients with the service for as long as they can benefit from it.

The format of the group can remain distinct and be offered repeatedly to new participants in time-limited sessions. For example, similar topics may be planned and covered for each session over the course of 8 weeks. An open-ended group that retains the same participants will need to create a new program format continuously in response to the group's development. The facilitator may find, for instance, that those who have been together for some time have less need to talk about the illness than do those who have not yet had the opportunity to discuss their concerns.

However, when a group is time limited it may seem that just as members have begun to know each other and have opened up, the session ends. The facilitator must be skilled in helping group members to "terminate"; that is, giving them the chance to acknowledge and react to the ending of the experience. Participants should also be referred elsewhere for ongoing services, although in most regions there are none available. Individuals who are still at a high level of functioning when the session ends may once again become isolated until the time that they need adult day care or other more intensive services. One hopes that there will eventually be many different program options available within the early stages of Alzheimer's disease. Then, perhaps a time-limited supportive discussion group could be followed up with an open-ended therapeutic activity (or other) format specific to those who have only mild impairment.

Disease progression is another important consideration. Participants in a time-limited group are likely to remain at a similar level of functioning throughout it. There is a greater chance in open-ended groups that the participants will advance in the illness, resulting in more variability in functioning among group members. The facilitator will then have the responsibility for determining when individuals are no longer appropriate for the group and helping them to "transition out." It can be uncomfortable for the participant, other group members, and the facilitator when it becomes apparent that someone is no longer benefiting from the program. For this reason, particularly in open-ended groups, continuous reassessment is necessary. One way a facilitator can allow for reassessment is to conduct a time-limited session followed by a break of several weeks during which the participants are reevaluated. Those participants who are able to continue have the option of enrolling in the next session. If others leave, space will then be available for new members. In this case, the facilitator will need to adjust his or her format to accommodate these changes and the varied needs of both new and continuing participants.

DURATION OF GROUP SESSIONS

The support group model discussed throughout this book is based on that of an 8-week session. However, other known groups have been conducted for other durations, including 10, 12, and 15 weeks.

Factors that go into the decision to have a time-limited group can also determine its optimum duration. The program format and resources and the availability of follow-up services in the region may influence the preferences and constraints under which the group operates.

It is always important to make sure that the participants understand the time-limited nature of the group. As mentioned previously, they should be reminded that the end is approaching before it occurs so that they have the opportunity to discuss and deal with the termination together. If handled appropriately, this will be a natural and nontraumatic part of the group process.

ASSESSING AND HANDLING CHANGES IN PARTICIPANTS' APPROPRIATENESS FOR THE GROUP

If the group is open ended, it is important that the facilitator monitor and reassess each participant's involvement over time. The need to address the progression of the illness in the context of discontinuing the program is a major concern for most who think of offering an open-ended group. Yet, situations like this can be managed with tact as well as practicality.

The groundwork can be laid during the initial selection and enrollment process (see Chapter 2). All group members and their families should be told that if an individual does not seem to be benefiting from or enjoying the meetings at a future point in time, reevaluation will be necessary. However, the facilitator can assure them that if this occurs, he or she will approach the participant and his or her family to ask for their input on the matter and make a decision *together* about continued participation. In addition, the determination will be based on the criteria and purpose of the group that should have been made explicit while interviewing potential members. Thus, the facilitator has already established an understanding of the policy and procedure before the group began.

Although it may seem difficult for a facilitator to reevaluate a participant who no longer is benefiting from a group, it is also difficult to have a participant who cannot comprehend or contribute to the group experience. That individual, the other group members, and the facilitator

90

would all be uncomfortable under such circumstances. Furthermore, because the facilitator has done his or her best to identify the individuals who acknowledge the illness and who have discussed it in the group, a basis exists for asking directly whether symptoms seem to be interfering with participation. However, forceful confrontation is never advisable. The participant may even be aware of increasing difficulty and may surprise the facilitator with the ability to articulate this.

The reevaluation process and discussion should take place outside of the group. All or some of the participant and caregiver interviews can be readministered and compared to initial results. Or, if the facilitator, the participant, and the caregiver are in immediate agreement about the need to discontinue, the facilitator can discuss the other resources (e.g., day programs, caregiver support groups) available of which they may not be aware. As mentioned previously, some regions are more likely than others to have services available for individuals who have just begun to have more moderate impairment or to have professionals in the field who can work with families to obtain new services. If there is no one else to provide these services, the facilitator may be called upon to help make the next care arrangements as a part of his or her service. This is similar to what the facilitator might do if he or she worked in a day program, and in-home or nursing home care needed to be explored.

In cases in which the participant and family do not agree with the facilitator's reassessment, he or she can try to resolve the differing perceptions. Talking through the issues, as well as the feelings involved in ending group participation, is likely to help all those involved reach a consensus. However, if the facilitator had discussed this in the initial agreement suggested above, he or she would have the prerogative to make the final decision. In most cases, the participants and families *will* agree with and/or accept the facilitator's judgment and be cooperative with the final decision.

If the individual with Alzheimer's disease is enrolled in a new program, the facilitator can explain to the group that a new service has been arranged and is likely to better suit this person's needs. The participant should have a chance to say anything he or she would like to say to other group members, including good-bye. Similarly, the other participants should be able to say anything they would like to say to this person. The facilitator may be surprised by the ability of the group members to do this and find that his or her own fears of how this would turn out are unfounded.

Remaining group participants may later want to express such feelings and concerns as missing the person who left or wondering if their own illnesses will also worsen. However, it is equally possible that no one will bring up these issues and a good facilitator should initiate discussion of these concerns.

If the facilitator finds these situations too difficult to handle or too emotionally distressing, outside supervision or consultation may be important to help manage these feelings.

OPEN VERSUS CLOSED ENROLLMENT

Once the participants have been selected to form a support group, the facilitator may want to take a break from interviewing other potential members. New referrals or inquiries can be put on a waiting list to be assessed and enrolled when space becomes available. Closing the enrollment period in this way allows group members to develop cohesiveness without constantly adjusting to new participants. This does create one risk, though, in that if several people decide to discontinue, the group may become too small.

However, if the facilitator interviews and enrolls participants on a continuous basis, the service will be accessible to more people. In addition, new personalities and ideas can keep the membership dynamic and interesting. Unfortunately, the facilitator will have the constant challenge of integrating and orienting recent arrivals with those who are already familiar and involved with the group.

One suggestion is to initially screen the first few people on the waiting list. Then, the facilitator can either add them if the membership drops too low during a session or have them join if a space opens during a break between time-limited sessions.

The decision should be tempered by the realization that the facilitator must be flexible in his or her expectations. The facilitator may lose members who decide the group is not right for them or who over time have a change in functioning. Also, those who do attend regularly might miss occasional meetings because of scheduling conflicts or other unavoidable circumstances.

MEETING ATTENDANCE, FREQUENCY, AND LENGTH

A group that is focused on intimate self-disclosure and supportive discussion functions best when there is minimal disruption. Members who commit to attending sessions regularly are more likely to sense that there is a stable foundation on which they can come to know and trust one another. If participants only attend intermittently it is more difficult to maintain continuity and structure and keep the format moving forward. In addition, the facilitator is better able to plan the content of each meeting and the resources if he or she knows who will be present for each session.

Groups most commonly meet weekly, biweekly, or monthly. Participants are often glad for the contact with others and enjoy having it on a weekly basis. This option can also potentially enhance a sense of routine and the chance to solidify relationships that have developed. Most importantly, perhaps, is the poignant reality that time is precious for people with Alzheimer's disease. The opportunity to meet frequently means that they will get as much as possible, as often as possible, out of the service.

The 8-week support group model described in this book is based on meetings that last for 1½ hours. In general, this allows an hour for the meeting and a half hour for the occasional late start or longer discussion. There is ample time to review or make announcements before and after each meeting. And, this extra half hour gives caregivers a bit more time between dropping off and picking up group participants.

It can be taxing for anyone to sit and talk intently with others for more than an hour. For individuals with Alzheimer's disease who have difficulty with concentration and attention, an hour is a particularly reasonable time frame. In the event that discussion ends or people get restless before the program is over, the facilitator may use brief activities or informal social time to occupy the time.

TIME AND PLACE OF MEETINGS

Support groups for people with Alzheimer's disease have been held in many different settings, including hospital-based day care programs, Alzheimer's Association offices, churches, colleges, and private clinicians' offices. Because individuals with early-stage Alzheimer's disease do not typically have unmanageable behavior problems, it is not necessary to meet in a locked facility. However, it is always wise for a facilitator to pay attention to the security of a potential setting. The facilitator will be responsible for the participants' safety and, in all likelihood, will have few people available to help supervise them.

When choosing the meeting site, the facilitator should ideally consider such factors as accessibility to wheelchairs, routes of public transportation, and ease of parking. It is also appropriate to have a pleasant and comfortable room environment that is easy to find and not institutional. However, deciding where to hold the meetings is likely to be ultimately determined by the space available or the agency sponsoring the group.

Late morning and early afternoon are times that have worked well for holding group meetings. However, there is no one time that is convenient for every participant and caregiver. Some individuals tire by late afternoon, while others become more confused at that time of day. One working family member might be able to transport a participant only in the evenings, while another does not like to go out at night. The facilitator might want to ask the participants and caregivers their preferences when setting up the group, and then try to accommodate the majority (along with his or her own schedule).

GROUP SIZE

An ideal size for a supportive discussion group is six to eight members. This size is not too big or too small and should be manageable in terms of monitoring each individual's participation level. If one or two people miss a particular session, decide to drop out, or are terminated from the program due to reassessment, there will still be an adequate number of remaining participants to continue. A group with more than eight members may become unwieldy, though, and members who are more quiet might be easily overlooked.

A group with as few as four members has also been successfully conducted. However, if there are fewer than four, the facilitator will certainly need at least one participant who is talkative. The group leader may also run into problems if several are absent the same day. Of course, this has also been known to happen in caregiver support groups, which results in the one or two people who are there getting personalized attention.

The decision about group size should be based on what is comfortable for the facilitator, as well as on the number of interested participants available and whether or not a cofacilitator will be available for assistance.

COMPOSITION OF THE MEMBERSHIP

The composition of the membership can be purposefully selected so that participants are either similar or diverse on any number of characteristics. For example, one group model has been developed specifically for people with Alzheimer's disease who are younger than age 65, and another is a "club" that only serves men with the illness. The rationale for these programs is that those of the same age group or gender may have more issues in common with one another and require a different approach from those of other or mixed gender or age groups. Although these innovative efforts are applauded, it is important to offer here an alternative perspective.

Group members who are heterogeneous in age, gender, ethnicity, and family structure can relate to one another and work together extremely well. Although participants in their 50s, for instance, are at different points in the life cycle from those older than 70, they all have the common need to cope with the many changes and losses that result from having Alzheimer's disease. Meeting others facing the same tasks is a great relief and usually enough of a basis on which to build relationships. In past support groups, each individual had a history, personality, and lifestyle prior to the illness, and each had a unique response to the onset of dementia, which could not be categorized by demographic attributes.

Therefore, it would seem that a valuable first step would be to have services more generally and widely available for individuals with early-stage Alzheimer's disease. Advocating for the needs of one group of individuals over another may jeopardize the broader aim at this point in time. Eventually, when all who seek groups can find one, specialized models can enrich the spectrum of service options.

If research is planned in conjunction with the group, a more homogeneous membership may be needed so that inferences are less subject to scientific error. In this case, selection criteria would be set up according to the study protocol, which may limit the pool of potential participants and require more time for recruitment.

Ultimately, what the facilitator decides for the composition of group membership will depend on his or her own areas of interest and expertise, the goals of the program effort, and the particular needs of potential clients who have come to the facilitator's attention.

ACCOMMODATING CULTURAL DIVERSITY

Because the understanding of the needs of people with early-stage Alzheimer's disease is still in its infancy, little is known about the appropriateness of various interventions for individuals with different cultural backgrounds.

It is important for facilitators to be sensitive to this issue in developing programs, as well as in adapting the techniques that are used. The primary support group model described in this book has served ethnically diverse participants within the same group. No noticeable differences have been perceived in interactions between these members, but there may have been subtle influences that were not apparent or explicit. There also may have been other participants who did not seek out a support group because they would not be comfortable in one. This might apply, for instance, to those for whom it is culturally "taboo" to discuss personal difficulties outside of the home.

However, a person cannot overgeneralize about culture-specific influences. Each participant and family has a distinct set of beliefs and traditions that may or may not be attributable to their cultural heritage. Furthermore, many people have roots in more than one ethnic population. In the ever-growing, mixing, and changing society, it may become less possible over time to ascribe a person's cultural identity in a simplistic or singular fashion.

It is crucial to study this area further through consulting with laypersons and professional members of as many ethnic communities as possible. Only then can existing services be modified and new ones developed that incorporate multicultural norms, values, customs, and languages. Trusted representatives of such communities can also assist with outreach and referral of people to services as well as with leading groups and training other facilitators.

CONCLUSION

The planning of a support group for individuals with early-stage Alzheimer's disease involves many decisions about its structure and membership. Various considerations have been identified for meeting time, place, duration, and frequency as well as for the heterogeneity of group participants. The need to monitor each group member over time and assist with transitions out of the program when appropriate has also been addressed.

5

Leading a
Support Group

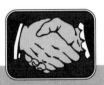

- Options for group format
- Anticipation and initiation of discussion topics
- Integrating the positive
- The facilitator's role and responsibilities
- Addressing the "hard truths" about Alzheimer's disease
- Unique group dynamics

Once the support group is underway, the facilitator will be responsible for shaping the format of meetings as well as the nature and content of discussion topics. The leader must also monitor and manage the many group dynamics that occur during the sessions. This chapter identifies specific roles and techniques that are instrumental in conducting groups for individuals with dementia.

OPTIONS FOR GROUP FORMAT

The approach outlined in this book is based on an 8-week, 1½-hour support group in which people with early-stage Alzheimer's disease share their feelings and experiences about coping with dementia. The facilitator provides structure and guidance but encourages the group members to actively engage and participate during each meeting. Discussion can be the sole format or it can be supplemented by other methods of stimulating interaction. For example, brief relaxation or stretching exercises may be used to begin or end meetings. A review of recent news clippings related to Alzheimer's disease keeps participants abreast of the latest research developments and can instill hope about the potential for future breakthroughs in treating and curing the illness. The reading of simple poetry or prose relevant to group topics may offer inspiration and alternative perspectives. Therapeutic reminiscence may occur when participants share their life histories in the context of all that is now changing for them.

Other program models focus less on discussion and more on recreational, social, vocational, or educational opportunities for people with early-stage Alzheimer's disease. Community outings, volunteer work, and creative arts projects are all examples of alternative group formats. In-depth information about a particular issue (e.g., legal planning) can be provided by a guest speaker who presents material in a structured way. Group participants can also take on educational projects, such as compiling their experiences for a newspaper article or a letter to policy makers.

The caregivers of group members may be involved in these programs for people with Alzheimer's disease or have a separate support group offered concurrently to them to focus on the early stages of caregiving. All of these various options are worthwhile, but beyond the scope of this book because each requires a different orientation and guidelines. One hopes that over time, many types of services will be available to people with early-stage Alzheimer's disease and their families, and information about developing them will be added to the existing literature.

ANTICIPATION AND INITIATION OF DISCUSSION TOPICS

The relationships established among the facilitator and group participants are the therapeutic fountainhead through which the group process flows. The facilitator sets the stage for self-disclosure girded by mutual respect by communicating interest, empathy, and acceptance.

Because each group and its leader have different personalities, it is important for facilitators to rely on their own intuition and style in conducting meetings. Members may be quite able to initiate topics and give input into the topics the facilitator suggests. Although the participants should be encouraged to do so, if necessary the group leader can be more directive in engaging them in discussion.

It is possible to anticipate a range of issues that will be significant to group participants. Specific concerns that were documented from actual group sessions can be found in the research summary (see Chapter 9). Such topics as understanding Alzheimer's disease; awareness of stigma around the illness; changes in lifelong activities, roles, and relationships; and the difficult balance between maintaining independence and facing increasing dependency are likely to be discussed in the group.

The sample session outline in Table 1 incorporates these and other important topics and can be used as a framework or guideline for the meetings in a time-limited session. This outline is for an 8-week program but can be reduced or expanded for sessions of varying lengths. Although such preparation is useful, the facilitator must be flexible in case what comes up is different from what was planned. For example, there may be overlap, issues that the facilitator did not anticipate, or areas requiring more or less time than the facilitator had allocated.

If the facilitator gives group participants and caregivers an outline of session topics, it is advisable to emphasize that it may change based on what occurs in the meetings. The facilitator may choose to rearrange the order of topics or subtopics or find that certain subjects depend on the level of intimacy that develops in the group.

INTEGRATING THE POSITIVE

Table 1 addresses the challenges people with Alzheimer's disease must face as well as the strengths they possess.

Table 1. Sample session outline for an 8-week support group for individuals with early-stage Alzheimer's disease

Week	Discussion topic	Issues
1	**Support group goals and ground rules**	Getting acquainted; explaining the purpose and format of the meetings; identifying participants' hopes and interests for the group; sharing what their experience has been
2	**Questions and concerns about memory loss**	Discussing how participants perceive their difficulties; providing information about Alzheimer's disease and other disorders based on what participants want to know (e.g., how a diagnosis is determined, what causes symptoms of dementia, what is being done to research and treat the illness)
3	**Coping with changes and feelings related to memory loss**	Acknowledging difficulties and changes in lifestyle; sharing specific coping strategies; dealing with stress and emotional reactions; nurturing the abilities that remain intact
4	**Adjusting to new situations**	Understanding the need for more assistance; finding ways to communicate effectively; adapting a different pace and set of expectations
5	**Relationships with family and friends**	Discussing the illness with family members and friends; adjusting to changes in roles and relationships; coping with others' reactions to symptoms

(continued)

Developing Support Groups for Individuals with Early-Stage Alzheimer's Disease: Planning, Implementation, and Evaluation by Robyn Yale   © 1995 Robyn Yale

Table 1. *(continued)*

Week	Discussion topic	Issues
6	**Wellness and optimism**	Finding activities that are manageable and pleasurable; maintaining good health and quality of life; recognizing the importance of mood and attitude
7	**Resources and support systems**	Finding sources of ongoing support and comfort; learning about the services available for all stages of Alzheimer's disease; understanding legal, financial, and health care planning considerations for the future
8	**Reviewing and ending the group experience**	Discussing what the group was like; expressing feelings about one another and about leaving; making plans for future group or other interactions
Optional:	**Inviting caregivers**	With the consent of the group, caregivers can be asked to join in the second half of the last session. Caregivers, participants, and the facilitator then have an opportunity to talk together in a large group about the experience. Feedback is useful to evaluate the program in general terms. The meeting could end with an informal social time in which plans are made for future contact or goodbyes are said.

Each group will find its own way of combining the positive and negative aspects of their life situations. Participants may interject serious and realistic discussion with optimism and humor. A skillful facilitator will always pay attention and contribute to the need for this balance and offer constructive ideas and strategies whenever possible.

It is likely that the group itself will become a positive experience for its members. The courage and camaraderie that are both created by and result from the group process should be acknowledged and praised often.

The goals of the support group discussed throughout this book are to share feelings as well as coping techniques. This dual focus helps to blend discussion of difficulties with problem-solving tactics. For example, in one actual session, participants shared a common frustration with losing or misplacing everyday items, such as jewelry and tools. They then generated a list of suggestions for reacting to these types of incidents. Although the ideas are brief and may seem simplistic, they represent a dozen alternatives for managing the stress that results from memory loss. However, it is important for a facilitator to point out to the participants that certain techniques might work better for some people than others or work more or less successfully for one person at different times. Figure 1 is a list of techniques for coping with memory loss generated by the members of a support group for individuals with early-stage dementia.

THE FACILITATOR'S
ROLE AND RESPONSIBILITIES

The facilitator's initial role is to create an atmosphere in which group participants feel comfortable and safe expressing themselves. Establishing norms or ground rules that everyone agrees on is an important first step. Repeat-

A CORNUCOPIA OF COPING TECHNIQUES

Take a break—admit you're upset.

Let it go.

Talk with someone to let out feelings and seek advice.

Laugh—look at the lighter side!

Know that misplaced items will turn up.

Use calendars, watches, and daily lists as memory aids.

Do not use a watch—takes away the pressure of rushing.

Be patient with yourself.

Allow more time to accomplish things—do not just give up!

Have kinder, more realistic expectations of yourself.

Acknowledge that things have changed.

Just do the best you can!

Figure 1. A list of coping techniques developed by support group participants in 1993. (Reprinted with permission of support group participants, 1993.)

ing these at the start of every meeting helps to focus attention on the group task and reinforce the understanding members have with one another. Figure 2 provides an introductory agreement that was originally developed for use with caregiver support groups but is just as useful in support groups for individuals with Alzheimer's disease. The facilitator strives to encourage group decision making about everything from format to topics, and foster interaction among participants. The extent to which the facilitator must intervene in and structure the group process depends on the nature and abilities of the members. For instance, the leader's role will be less active if most individuals are eager to talk than it will if most of them are reserved.

As in any group setting, the leader monitors the level of each individual's participation. Members who are quiet and those with more cognitive impairment may need to be drawn out with direct and special attention from the facilitator. Limits should also be set on participants who tend to dominate the discussion. A participant's cognitive impairment may also require the facilitator to introduce only one question or idea at a time and to be very concrete and specific in reframing or restating themes to sustain the flow of conversation. The leader must also keep the meeting on track if it digresses and provide explanations and reassurance if anxiety or confusion arises.

The facilitator will have to be prepared for each session and yet be flexible enough to adapt to unplanned directions that might emerge. In addition, a facilitator must remember that it will take time to get to know group members and to become experienced with this intervention. There is no way to prepare a group leader for the myriad of subjects and situations to which he or she may be called on to respond. If facilitators have a solid back-

SUPPORT GROUP
OUR PLEDGE
TO EACH OTHER

We have the right to silence; no one has to talk.

We agree to confidentiality; personal information is not discussed outside the group.

We share our time together; we give everyone time to talk.

We are considerate of each other; we listen carefully to others.

We affirm how we feel; it's okay to cry and to laugh.

We are flexible in meeting needs; let us know what you need and how best to serve you.

We begin and end on time.

Used with permission—Alzheimer's Association, Greater San Francisco Bay Area Chapter.

SUPPORT GROUP
OUR
PURPOSE AND GOALS

We gather to allow people touched by Alzheimer's disease and other related disorders to be together in a caring and understanding environment.

To learn more about Alzheimer's disease and related disorders.

To share our experiences.

To express our feelings.

To learn about helpful resources.

To hear about advances in research and advocacy.

To remember that laughter, taking care of ourselves, and planning for the future are essential for our well-being.

To help others who are going where we have been.

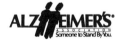

Figure 2. A support group agreement that can be repeated at the beginning of every support group meeting.

ground in caring for people with dementia and basic group work skills (and their hearts are in the right place), they should be confident in relying on their own intuition and judgment.

ADDRESSING THE "HARD TRUTHS" ABOUT ALZHEIMER'S DISEASE

Another primary aspect of the facilitator's role is to be a resource person for group participants. Group leaders should maintain a thorough and ongoing knowledge base about the illness and have updated information and resources available.

Unfortunately, virtually all of the lay and professional literature about Alzheimer's disease focuses on its long-term course and symptoms. A typical article about Alzheimer's disease reads that of the 4 million Americans affected by Alzheimer's disease, most will ultimately become unable to care for themselves or to recognize loved ones and will die in nursing homes. Although these statements may be true, other equally important truths have been overlooked. New printed materials for people with early-stage Alzheimer's disease and their caregivers are urgently needed to offer an additional perspective. Articles and literature should report that people who are diagnosed with Alzheimer's disease when they have only mild impairment may maintain good health and functioning for several years. It is also important to convey that the rate and impact of decline differs for each individual because many are able to adjust well to new ways of living even as they face the uncertainty of the future.

Similarly, the group facilitator is challenged to both educate the participants about the realities of the illness *and* emphasize each individual's existing abilities and capabilities. Guidance around integrating the two will come from the group participants themselves. The following synopsis of an actual session demonstrates this:

Mr. J: I've been thinking about how things might go for me. Do any of you ever worry about what will happen if you get worse?

Mr. R: I sometimes wonder what it would be like if I become unable to speak.

Mr. H: Well I'm concerned about those things, but I try not to dwell on them....I feel good now, and I take each day as it comes.

Mrs. T: That's a smart way to look at it. After all, we have to go on living.

One might expect that a range of other emotions may also be expressed during this interchange, such as fear, anger, denial, and despair. (See Chapters 5 and 6 for suggestions about handling these reactions.) The point of the illustration above is that the group is a place where individuals can ask their questions and acknowledge their feelings and concerns while also striving to cope successfully with the illness.

The facilitator must remember that he or she has carefully selected group participants who do not usually deny their symptoms and who want to learn and talk about Alzheimer's disease. Normally, information regarding a health condition (e.g., cancer, heart disease) is provided directly to the individuals who receive these diagnoses. A general prognosis, suggestions for self-care, and planning considerations are explained by physicians, health and social service agencies, and leaders of disease-specific support groups. However, professionals typically have not had the same protocol with people who have early-stage Alzheimer's disease. Although discomfort is understandable, group facilitators and other providers are advised to examine their own issues and skills in this area and to obtain support as needed. Group participants are likely to welcome news of the services available in their communities. One approach that works well is to offer a list of local resources covering areas like day programs, elder law specialists, medical research centers, caregiver support groups, and Alzheimer's Association telephone helplines. A facilitator can introduce available services by saying, "No one can predict how each individual will be affected by Alzheimer's disease as time passes. It is known that it is progressive, but the timing and rate of this are different for each person. Some people remain quite healthy for long periods of time; some experience worsening symptoms of dementia; and some are affected by other illnesses or die of natural causes rather than reaching late-stage Alzheimer's disease. Therefore, you may or may not use all of the services on this list, but it is good to know about them."

Education can be provided at the same time by the facilitator saying, for example, "All of us should make legal and financial arrangements for the future (e.g., drafting a will) because we never know what might befall us. When an illness like Alzheimer's disease strikes, this becomes particularly important. It is best to consult with an attorney who has special expertise in this aspect of law and can explain the issues and options to you."

Group participants should be encouraged to share their knowledge and experiences with one another. The facilitator can engage the group by asking, "Have any of you ever used any of these services? Can you tell us about it? What was it like? Was it helpful to you?" Interactions between members in actual group sessions can be found in the research summary in Chapter 9.

UNIQUE GROUP DYNAMICS

As group members become cohesive and work toward common goals, they are influenced by a variety of interpersonal dynamics. The facilitator must be aware of this natural developmental process and intervene as necessary to keep the group environment safe and under control. In any group setting there are likely to be similar issues requiring attention, such as certain people interrupting or dominating the conversation. Additional skills are needed to manage the distinctive characteristics of group work with people who have cognitive impairment.

Below are some challenges that may emerge in the group as well as suggested techniques and examples a facilitator needs to work through each situation. This list can be used as a training tool for facilitators to anticipate potential disruptions and to practice handling these and other phenomena. The role plays in Chapter 8 incorporate much of what follows into situations that can be further rehearsed and discussed.

A facilitator must remember that the more care he or she takes to select only those participants with high levels of functioning, the less likely he or she is to experience the challenges illustrated below. However, it is good to be familiar with and prepared for the "unexpected." In fact, the onset of increased memory loss, communication problems, or behavior problems may signal a change in status and the need to reevaluate appropriateness for the group.

Group Process Issues

1. **Memory impairment—forgetfulness, short attention span**
   Techniques: Refocus, repeat, and reassure.
   Provide structure and consistency.

115

Point out commonalities among members and between situations within and outside of group.

Example: A participant becomes confused about the focus of the group and periodically says things like, "What are we doing here?" Rather than let this disrupt the meeting, the facilitator can respond in a calm and tactful way by saying, "It's okay that you've forgotten—that's exactly what this support group focuses on! Do others of you experience memory loss at home or in social situations? What do you do when that happens?"

2. **Communication deficits—difficulty finding and/or understanding words**

   Techniques: Simplify language and speaking style.

   Allow silence and extra time to respond.

   Ask permission to assist their self-expression.

   Be aware of nonverbal messages.

   Respond to the underlying feelings when words are not understood.

   Example: A participant relating an anecdote is suddenly unable to complete a sentence and exclaims, "Oh, !*@#! I can't find the...." The facilitator can respond with, "It must be frustrating when you have trouble speaking—take your time. Is it okay if I review what I understood you to say so far?...[if so] We were talking about friendships, and you were just telling us about your former business partner. Was there something special about that relationship?"

3. **Behavior problems—unpredictable or inappropriate behavior**

   Techniques: Stay calm and in control.

Use diversion or breaks.

Look for the underlying reason for the behavior.

Example: A participant gets up while someone else is talking and walks toward the door saying, "I have to leave now." The facilitator asks what this person is concerned about and he answers, "I'd like to find my wife. She may not know where I am." The leader reassures him, "Your wife knows to come here to pick you up at 2:30—that's about 10 minutes from now. You'd better stick around so you don't miss her." If the participant becomes more agitated, he could be accompanied for a short walk down the hall and back—he may be ready for a stretch. (This is also a good example of the help a cofacilitator can provide.)

Participants in the early stages of Alzheimer's disease who are willing and able to be in the group are not likely to exhibit difficult behavior problems. If the facilitator has concerns about clinical symptoms of depression, anxiety, or psychosis co-existing with dementia, psychiatric assessment should be recommended to family members to see if medication or other forms of treatment are warranted.

4. **Emotional reactions—intense feelings about the subject matter**

   Techniques: Accept, "normalize," and empathize.

   Respect each person's style and limits.

   Refer for psychiatric consultation, if appropriate.

   Integrate the positive into the discussion.

   Example: During a discussion about becoming more dependent on others for assistance, a participant begins to cry, saying, "I'm so upset! I've always taken care of everything myself!" The facilitator engages others to share how they have reacted to increasing dependence, allowing and validating expressed feelings of anger and sadness. The facilitator can also ask, "Although these are difficult adjustments, has anyone felt relieved to have less responsibility—say, for keeping track of finances? Has the help you've gotten in any areas made things easier for you?"

Even if the facilitator takes care to select participants who usually acknowledge their condition, some people intermittently cope with denial. As described in Chapter 2, a good approach is to back off and allow the person to keep this defense intact. Therefore, if in this example the participant says, "I don't have any problems that I need help with," the facilitator can reply, "Oh, I see. Does anyone else have experiences to share?"

Gentle peer support and encouragement often come from other participants, who have been noted to say things such as, "You might feel better if you admit it—besides, why would you want to come here if you aren't going through these things?" If conveyed with compassion and sensitivity, such feedback from other participants can be very effective in helping individuals to open up. There is also a difference between denying and forgetting that one has a diagnosis of Alzheimer's disease. The latter is handled differently in terms of carefully reminding individuals that they are in the group because they have memory problems.

The facilitator's skill will be called upon, though, to assist members in maintaining boundaries when necessary. That is, no one should be subjected to prolonged confrontation or bombardment from others.

Of course, if a stance of denial persists, the facilitator may want to look at whether staying in the group is appropriate for this person.

5. **Fluctuating capacity—moods and abilities vary over time**
   Techniques: Interpret changes as being caused by the disease process.
   Acknowledge losses, including termination of group and/or individual members.

Example: A participant's cognition has declined over the course of the session and she, her husband, and the facilitator have decided together that she should no longer return. On her last day in attendance, the leader announces, "Mrs. S. will not be coming to the group anymore. Although we hate to see her go, she will be attending the Alzheimer's day program near her home, which has a fine reputation for their specialized staff and activities. Sometimes a comprehensive center like that can better meet the special needs of people with memory loss. I'd like to give Mrs. S. a chance to say good-bye to this group, and for all of you to wish her well today." This allows both the participant leaving and the other group members to bring closure to their relationships and to have changes in attendance be acknowledged and explained.

6. **Participant's reaction to the facilitator—distinguishing transference, reminiscence, and disorientation**
   Techniques: Facilitate therapeutic grief work.
   Gently reorient the participants to the here-and-now.
   Be aware of the relationship with each participant.

119

Example: During a discussion of family life, a participant points to the group leader and says to the other participants, "This is my daughter." The facilitator is not sure whether the participant is reacting to her on a psychological level, is reminded of her daughter by powerful memories that have been stirred, or is mistaking the present for another time or place. An appropriate response would be, "We have been talking in our support group today about family members, and this has made you think of your daughter. Perhaps I also remind you of her. Would you like to tell us about her?

7. **Facilitator's reaction to the participants—dealing with difficult questions and situations**
   Techniques: Keep expectations of "treatment" realistic.

   Be aware of and seek support for personal issues and feelings.

Example: The facilitator's father has had Alzheimer's disease for 6 years and is now experiencing increasing decline. In one group session covering recent medical advances, a participant asks, "If they are doing so much research these days, how come they still don't know how to beat this disease?" The group leader, having heard his own father say similar things in the past, is filled with feelings of helplessness and despair. However, he is able to recognize that although he cannot offer these participants a cure, he has provided them with an enriching experience during this early point in the disease course. He replies, "That's a good question....We can only hope that all the work that has been done is leading scientists closer to the answers. In the meantime, as we talk about in our group, good physical and mental health will help to keep everyone at his or her best for as long as possible."

Later that day, the facilitator resolves to seek out clinical supervision, peer consultation, or individual therapy to tend to his own emotional needs because of his father's illness. By doing so, he will be better able to separate his personal and professional selves, thereby enhancing his functioning in and enjoyment of the support group for individuals with dementia.

CONCLUSION

A facilitator must use specialized skills and techniques in leading a support group for individuals with Alzheimer's disease. The topics discussed, interactions between participants, and unique group dynamics all pose continual challenges for the group leader. However, these responsibilities are manageable and it is possible to balance acknowledgment of the difficulties participants experience with emphasis on their strengths.

6

ADMINISTERING AND EVALUATING A SUPPORT GROUP

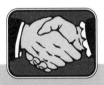

- Public relations with the service community and media
- Sample materials for outreach and participant recruitment
- Group fees
- Transportation of participants
- The limits of liability
- Emergency protocol
- Documentation of client and program characteristics
- Recording group sessions
- Observing and analyzing group sessions
- Evaluating the program

S upport groups for individuals with early-stage Alzheimer's disease are still relatively new and unstudied. Close monitoring is critical for purposes of accountability as is continuous feedback from which to refine the program. This chapter discusses administrative areas such as publicity, fees, and reporting and provides reproducible forms that may be used to observe and evaluate group sessions.

PUBLIC RELATIONS WITH
THE SERVICE COMMUNITY AND MEDIA

Staggering statistics on the incidence and prevalence of Alzheimer's disease and advances in detecting it make it reasonable to assume that many individuals with dementia are being diagnosed early enough in the illness to be appropriate for a support group. It is advisable for the person seeking participants (usually the facilitator) to "cast a wide net" in recruiting efforts and pursue several avenues simultaneously in order to find individuals with early-stage Alzheimer's disease. Plenty of time must be allowed (i.e., up to several months) for publicizing the service, as well as for conducting the intensive participant selection process described in Chapter 2.

One primary source of referrals is the local network of service providers for individuals with dementia and their families. Caregiver support group leaders and agencies (e.g., diagnostic, day care, resource centers) should be glad to hear about the support group because often they come in contact with individuals in the early stages of Alzheimer's disease and their families, but they have no services specifically available for them. Mailing a flyer, listing the group in newsletters for professionals and clients, and speaking directly with key agency staff are all good ways for the facilitator to make these individuals and their families aware of his or her new program.

Unfortunately, many communities have no central agency or professional responsible for assisting clients in following through on referrals to programs, and this is a large service gap. Strengthening the ties between the facilitator's group service for people with early-stage Alzheimer's disease and providers of other services may go a long way toward reducing this type of fragmentation. Future access to resources and support as the disease progresses may also be enhanced if the local, mutual referral mechanism is improved.

The facilitator might consider holding a meeting for key service providers in which he or she talks about the needs of the community and introduces them to the group project. From this meeting, a consortium can be organized whose focus of activity is to improve service coordination.

Another suggestion for finding group participants is to tap into the larger community of services for older people who are healthy, such as senior centers and retirement facilities. After all, the early stages of dementia usually affect people who are otherwise healthy (physically and mentally) and whose onset of cognitive impairment is slow and subtle. They may, for instance, be living alone and functioning relatively well, or they may need more supervision and socialization but not realize or accept that they do. Because there can be surprisingly little interaction between general providers of services for older people and providers of services specifically for individuals with dementia, the facilitator can make efforts to establish relationships by directly contacting the former through letters, telephone calls, and site visits.

The media is an invaluable tool for finding group participants. Because individuals with early-stage dementia are neither all elderly nor all in contact with agencies, newspaper articles and radio spots can be targeted to the general public as well as more strategically to seniors. Public service announcements on the radio, on television, or in newspapers are often effective. Although listing or advertising the group may make it visible, the facilitator is more likely to capture the attention of potential participants by explaining and humanizing the goals of the program. The way in which the group is described may make a difference in the response that is received. Focusing more on support and coping skills and less on disability may even lead individuals who have the illness to personally contact the facilitator about their interest.

This type of perspective on early-stage Alzheimer's disease is greatly needed to educate both the general public and many health care providers. If mainstream and professional media reflect values of discussing the disease openly and seeking to maintain a high quality of life for as long as possible, the stigma and stereotypes about people with dementia will ultimately be challenged. The facilitator or agency sponsoring the group should consider producing a program brochure, developing fact sheets or pamphlets, or appearing on a radio talk show as a few ways to combine the marketing and educational efforts of the support group.

It is important for a facilitator to remember that although he or she wants to inform people and generate interest about the group, the need for balance between publicity and program development must be considered. If demand for the service greatly exceeds the group's capacity, individuals may end up on waiting lists with their future appropriateness for the group a major uncertainty. However, a big response continues to demonstrate the need for more services to become available. One hopes that the amount and type of early-stage programs that exist will eventually be greatly increased.

SAMPLE MATERIALS FOR OUTREACH AND PARTICIPANT RECRUITMENT

There are many different possible formats for resource and publicity materials. Three examples are presented below.

Newsletters

An excellent resource in which to publicize a newly formed support group is an Alzheimer's Association chapter newsletter, which is sent to professionals as well as individuals with Alzheimer's disease and their families. Figure 1 appeared in one such newsletter to encourage caregivers to attend support groups. There is actually not one word or idea in Figure 1 that cannot be applied equally to individuals with Alzheimer's disease. This type of item can be used, then, to educate and entice people with early-stage Alzheimer's disease to participate in support groups as well.

Flyers

Flyers are an effective way to spread the news about a support group. Figure 2 is a sample of a flyer sent to families and service providers publicizing a local support group for individuals with dementia. The more specific the facilitator can be about particular selection criteria, the less like-

Experience and friendship can give us strength to cope with the tragedy of Alzheimer's disease. We learn from each other and, most importantly, we learn we are not alone. A support group is...

- A place to go for specialized information about your particular problem.
- A group of special friends who are good listeners and care about you.
- An inexpensive, sharing experience.
- A place to give and receive strength and understanding.
- A place to receive reassurance, comfort, friendship, and social support.
- People like yourself who share a common problem or interest.
- A place where you can laugh at the ridiculous side of tragedy without being considered "odd" or "unfeeling."
- A gathering attended by people who have a common bond: the challenge of coping with a particularly difficult experience.

Used with permission—Alzheimer's
Association, Akron, Ohio Chapter

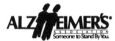

Figure 1. Newsletters are an excellent means for publicizing a support group. This is an example of a notice for a support group in an Alzheimer's Association Newsletter.

ly he or she is to be bombarded by calls from people who are not appropriate for the group.

Press Releases

Figure 3 is a press release developed during recruitment for the research study described in Chapter 9. As a result of the press release, the project was written up in many lo-

---

Marin Alzheimer's Association is offering
A NEW SUPPORT GROUP FOR INDIVIDUALS WITH
EARLY-STAGE ALZHEIMER'S DISEASE—WITH OPTIONAL,
SEPARATE GROUP FOR FAMILY MEMBERS

- Sessions for individuals with Alzheimer's disease will combine education and support to enhance understanding of and coping with the illness.
- Sessions for family members will occur separately (but at the same time) to address questions and concerns specific to mild dementia.
- The 8 weekly meetings will be free of charge and run every Friday beginning February 4 and ending March 25, 1994, from 1:00 p.m.–2:30 p.m. in San Rafael.
- Facilitators will be Robyn Yale and Barbara Khurana, qualified professionals experienced in working with people with Alzheimer's disease.

We are seeking individuals with a physician's diagnosis of dementia, who have been told of and at least occasionally acknowledge the illness, have good communication and social skills, and would like to be in the group.

Potential participants (and/or family members):
Please call the Marin Alzheimer's Association office
(415) 472-4340 to set up an interview.

**Used with permission—Alzheimer's
Association, Marin County Chapter**

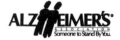

Figure 2. An example of a flyer used to publicize a support group.

cal newspapers and newsletters. These articles were responsible for a large percentage of inquiries about the support group, some of which came from individuals with Alzheimer's disease who had read about the group in the morning paper.

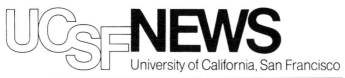

University of California, San Francisco

513 Parnassus Avenue Room S101
San Francisco, CA 94143-0462
(415) 476-2557
FAX (415) 665-8668

Carol Fox, News Director
Source: Bill Gordon (415) 476-2557

FOR IMMEDIATE RELEASE
February 3, 1992

**UCSF ALZHEIMER CENTER OFFERS PEER SUPPORT GROUPS
FOR PATIENTS IN EARLY STAGES OF DISEASE**

A new UC San Francisco program will allow patients in the early stages of Alzheimer's Disease to turn to each other for understanding and information.

Peer support groups will be offered by the UCSF Memory Clinic and Alzheimer Center to study how patients respond upon learning of their diagnosis, explore the issues they confront early in the course of the disease, and determine whether such groups can help them deal with the problems that emerge.

"There are many support groups for caregivers of Alzheimer's patients but very few groups for the patients. We want to offer patients an opportunity to learn about their disease and talk to others in the same situation," said Robyn Yale, a licensed clinical social worker at the Alzheimer Center and facilitator of the groups.

Two support groups of six to eight members each will meet weekly for two months starting in March. Volunteers are being sought for the pilot study, funded by the National Alzheimer's Association. Those interested in participating in the study should contact the UCSF Alzheimer Center at (415) 476-7606.

"Patients in the early stages of Alzheimer's disease often can communicate well enough to talk about the illness, the

(continued)

Figure 3. A press release used to publicize the support group for the research study in Chapter 9.

Figure 3. *(continued)*

changes it has caused in their lives, and the ways they and their families deal with these changes," Yale said.

"But Alzheimer's patients and their families typically find few services available to assist them between the time of diagnosis and the time at which they require more comprehensive care," Yale said. In many cases, patients rarely even hear the term "Alzheimer's disease" during this period, which can extend for several years.

Alzheimer's disease is a progressive, degenerative disease of the brain which results in impaired memory, thinking, and behavior. It affects an estimated 4 million American adults.

Project coordinators want to learn whether participation in the support groups helps the patients to feel less isolated, reduces their families' sense of burden, and encourages patients and their families to plan together for the future. Patients and their families also can learn earlier on about community resources in such areas as legal planning, counseling, or long-term care.

Those interested in participating in the study must have received a diagnosis of probable Alzheimer's disease within the past year. Patients must be able and willing to participate in a support group and must not have other significant medical or psychiatric conditions. Participants also must have a caregiver who is willing to be interviewed.

Study coordinators include Joseph C. Barbaccia, MD, UCSF professor of Family and Community Medicine and medical director of the Alzheimer Center, and Linda S. Mitteness, PhD, UCSF associate professor of medical anthropology.

The Memory Clinic and Alzheimer Center operates as an outpatient clinic of UCSF's Langley Porter Psychiatric Institute, providing comprehensive evaluations for people experiencing confusion and memory loss. Medical, psychiatric, neuropsychological, social, and nursing assessments are combined to diagnose patients and make recommendations for their care.

The UCSF Alzheimer Center is one of nine designated by the California Department of Health Services to provide diagnostic services, offer education and training, and conduct research in the field of Alzheimer's disease.

GROUP FEES

The issue of whether to charge a fee for the group depends on factors that include who is sponsoring it, the structure and philosophy of the program, and what resources are available. Of course, a service that is free or low cost is always preferable from the "consumer's" point of view, especially in light of other necessary health care expenses. Offering services at no cost may also be part of an agency's mission or policy statement, as has been the case with caregiver support groups provided by the Alzheimer's Association.

However, there is consensus among many people who work in the Alzheimer's disease field that, given the level of skill required, support groups for individuals with dementia should be facilitated by professionals rather than laypersons. Chapter 3 has more information on the recommended qualifications of a group facilitator. Finding professionals who are willing and able to volunteer their time so that groups can be free of charge is likely to be difficult. Therefore, as with any new program effort, diverse sources of funding may be necessary in order to cover staffing and overhead expenses. Options in addition to or in lieu of increasing agency budgets include grants, donations, and fund-raising events. Groups can also be conducted by licensed clinicians in private practice who structure the group as "therapy" and submit claims for insurance reimbursement.

There is no standard fee for support groups for people with dementia. Rates vary by type of service, provider or source, and region. Other factors include session length and costs, such as meeting space and monetary compensation for facilitators. Some programs have offered free sessions for several months and as it became more established over time started to charge $5 or $10 for each meeting. Other groups charge as much as $15 and $20 per meeting. Regardless of what is decided, it is always important to consider subsidizing or having a sliding fee scale available for people with limited financial resources.

TRANSPORTATION OF PARTICIPANTS

It would be ideal if all providers had the resources to offer transportation to and from group meetings. In most cases, though, this will not be possible because there are typically not enough community transportation or casework services available, especially for something that as a rule would not be deemed "medically necessary." In rural areas in particular, lack of transportation can be a major barrier to service utilization.

A wise policy for a facilitator is to have someone, usually a family member, commit to bringing participants to the group and supervising them before and after the meetings. For example, it would not be advisable to have a caregiver drop a participant off in front of the building or have him or her wait alone outside to be picked up. Although most participants might be perfectly capable in these situations, it is better to take extra precautions. If someone is more confused than usual on a given day, he or she may be at risk of getting hurt or lost in relatively unfamiliar surroundings.

Some group participants may actually be able to get to and from meetings independently or via public transportation. Others might live alone or may not have a family to drive them. It is unfortunate when someone who is otherwise right for the group is unable to participate because there is no one to escort him or her to the sessions. However, the facilitator must decide what is the most comfortable and may rightfully choose not to assume sole responsibility for whether the participants safely arrive and return home from meetings.

THE LIMITS OF LIABILITY

The research project reported on in Chapter 9 required review by a university "Human Subjects Committee." The protocol included signing a "Consent to Participate in Research" form that explained the study's purpose, potential risks, and benefits. The issues covered were important and have been adapted in this book into a format that can be used for everyday practice.

The recommended combination of well-screened participants, skilled facilitators, and a safe environment should result in the group running smoothly 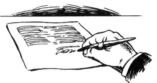 and without any major crises. However, to err on the side of caution, the facilitator may want to make any concerns about *unanticipated* events explicitly known. This is a relatively new mental health intervention and its effectiveness has not yet been extensively studied. There is always some degree of vigilance required in any program setting to ensure the physical safety and supervision of individuals with Alzheimer's disease. A contract acknowledging the limits of professional knowledge and responsibility can help clarify these issues.

The facilitator or agency sponsoring the group may choose to develop a brochure for marketing purposes and a separate concise and specific agreement addressing liability issues. Or, as in Figure 4, a program description may be combined with an enrollment agreement that also acts as a "waiver of liability." Although this type of agreement is

SUPPORT GROUP FOR
INDIVIDUALS WITH EARLY-STAGE DEMENTIA

Program Description & Agreement

The Alzheimer's Association is pleased to offer this new program specially designed for individuals in the early stages of Alzheimer's disease or a related disorder. It provides an opportunity for those with mild memory loss to meet others who are experiencing similar difficulties and exchange information and support in group discussions.

The topic of memory impairment, including references to Alzheimer's disease and dementia, will naturally be a part of the group experience. For this reason, we hope to enroll only participants who are willing and able to share their feelings and experiences. Although this is a relatively new approach for people with early-stage dementia, initial findings have been positive, in terms of such benefits as decreased isolation, improved mood, and increased self-esteem.

Participants (and their caregivers) will be interviewed prior to enrollment to determine suitability for the group and provide background information. Specific information shared in these interviews and in group sessions will be considered confidential. However, general information about discussion topics and each participant's contribution to the group will be conveyed to caregivers. All clients will be asked to assist the Alzheimer's Association in evaluating the program after the final session.

Participants who sign below agree to attend and become involved in the program. Caregivers who sign below will not attend group meetings but agree to designate or serve as a contact person, take responsibility for the participant's safe transport to and from the program, and notify the facilitator about any change in arrangements. Caregivers are welcome to call the Association for information about other services available to them, such as caregiver support groups and educational programs.

(continued)

Figure 4. An example of a program description and enrollment agreement among the participant, caregiver, and facilitator or agency sponsoring the group.

136

Figure 4. *(continued)*

The 8 weekly, 1½-hour sessions will be facilitated by one licensed clinical social worker on contract and one volunteer with our agency. Both have experience in the field of dementia care and have received additional orientation and training to conduct this group. The meetings will be held in a community agency setting that is not secured or locked.

As a condition of enrollment, the group facilitators are hereby authorized in the event of an emergency to obtain any medical or other assistance necessary for the care of the participant until such time as his or her family can be contacted. Furthermore, the caregiver signing below agrees to assume all risks and hazards that are incidental to the conduct of this activity and agrees to absolve, release, indemnify, and hold harmless the Alzheimer's Association and the organizers and facilitators of this activity of any and all legal responsibilities.

_____   _____
Participant   Association representative

_____   _____
Caregiver   Date

Used with permission. This document was developed by the author and amended by the Alzheimer's Association, Greater San Francisco Bay Area Chapter

not likely to be legally binding, it does establish a basis of understanding among the group participants and their families. Each group facilitator and/or sponsoring agency is also strongly encouraged to have professional liability insurance. This may already be in place if the facilitator is currently conducting caregiver support groups.

Figure 4 is an example that can be adapted to fit each facilitator's own style and setting. This example contains considerations that may or may not apply for each facilitator, including transportation, confidentiality, and medical emergencies. The facilitator might also have things to add, such as asking permission to videotape sessions. If further suggestions or formal guidance is needed, the document can be reviewed by a lawyer.

EMERGENCY PROTOCOL

Before beginning a group, it is advisable for a facilitator to think through potential emergencies that might arise and delineate procedures for how he or she would handle them. Even in the best of circumstances, unforeseen events not resulting from negligence can occur. This should not need to unduly alarm the facilitator, because most of it (if it occurs at all) can be dealt with by good planning and common sense.

Staffing of the group is one important consideration. Will there be a cofacilitator or volunteer present who can assist the facilitator in the event of an emergency? If not, is the group in a setting where the facilitator can ask for the help of someone in a nearby office? Will this person know how to calm and relate to the other participants with Alzheimer's disease? Is there a telephone accessible for calling 911?

Medical conditions are another area for precaution. Does the intake form cover each participant's health status, as well as his or her doctors and any medication he or she is taking? Are the names and telephone numbers of more than one family contact person accessible? Is it appropriate to ask a physician that the facilitator or the sponsoring agency works with if he or she can be called in an emergency? Is the location of the closest hospital known?

Psychiatric emergencies are also a remote possibility. Will the facilitator be able to handle a participant who unexpectedly becomes agitated or combative? Who will stay with the group participants if the facilitator needs to take this person from the room? Is there backup in place for seeking consultation from psychiatric professionals? The last situation that comes to mind is what to do if a participant becomes suicidal in the group because he or she has Alzheimer's disease. This question is asked often by providers who are contemplating offering support groups, and the concern is legitimate. (It also underscores the need for facilitators to be qualified professionals who can be competent in these situations, as discussed in Chapter 3.)

The facilitator must be skilled in the standard means of assessing the level of depression and the severity of suicidal ideation. The facilitator must use his or her clinical judgment—the first step might be to see how the individual responds to the other participants who provide support and perspective in the session. Even if this person's mood lifts, though, it is imperative that the facilitator probes further after the meeting to determine whether the participant feels safe. The facilitator can also then ask permission to discuss the situation with the caregiver who comes to pick up the participant. The facilitator, participant, and caregiver should talk about the issues and make a plan together, including referrals for suicide prevention and mental health treatment. (See also Chapter 7 on reporting laws.) If the facilitator does not believe he or she is qualified or prepared to deal with a situation like this, he or she should seek education and training regarding it.

Although it is unpleasant to think of these situations happening, it is better to anticipate and plan for them than to be caught unaware if they do. Although crises can occur anytime and anywhere, they are largely not insurmountable. Furthermore, the group may even be helping to prevent other crises from occurring. For example, a support group may be invaluable to those people who are depressed because they do not understand what is happening to them or have no one to talk to about it. In fact, group support from peers can *improve* the participants' emotional health (as discussed in the self-reports of participants and caregivers in Chapter 9).

DOCUMENTATION OF CLIENT AND PROGRAM CHARACTERISTICS

There are several good reasons for a facilitator to collect basic data on the client population and on his or her new program. As discussed previously, the concept of services specific to the needs of people with early-stage dementia is still relatively new. In most regions, little attention has been paid to the idea, and few if any funds have been allocated to it. Program development may be slowed by the need for multilevel policy changes, which typically require justification in terms of definitions and "numbers." Ongoing reporting is often necessary to sustain fledgling efforts.

The more that pioneering facilitators record their experiences, the more precisely these clients with early-stage dementia will come to be identified and understood. This in turn will supply agency boards of directors, public and private funding sources, policy makers, and other "powers that be" with the information they will request to move forward in this area. Advocacy, education, outreach, research, and service efforts can be better shaped by continued documentation and analysis of the following areas:

• Who are these participants and families?
• What prompts these individuals to seek support?

- Which program format suits a particular type of person and level of functioning?
- What benefits of programs are measured and/or reported?
- What capabilities and limitations define the "early stages"?
- Who is *not* appropriate for such services, and how can this be easily determined?
- What facilitates or impedes the use of available services?
- What supplemental services are sought or utilized?

It would be ideal if data collection were uniform, similar to what is done in multisite diagnostic, resource, and research centers, and designed fairly simply as a routine part of the group participant screening process. For example, the facilitator can use the answers on the intake form (see Chapter 2) to understand and record instances in which selection criteria were not met and reasons participants who could be accepted chose not to be in the group. This type of information clarifies the characteristics favorable for referral to support groups for people with early-stage Alzheimer's disease, as well as sheds light on concurrent unmet service needs. Unmet service needs may include a participant who has met the screening criteria but has no way to get to the group meetings. Or, the group may be full but a waiting list maintained to demonstrate the demand for service expansion.

The intake form also records who referred the participants to the group. This is useful in examining what outreach efforts were most effective and what efforts can be emphasized and strengthened in future recruiting efforts.

A more comprehensive picture of any agency's client base is obtained through tabulation of intakes, and those who are not appropriate for this particular service can be readily referred to other community resources.

RECORDING GROUP SESSIONS

There are pros and cons to recording group sessions. A recorded session can be useful for review to analyze the group process, to study the need to refine facilitation techniques, and to educate and train others interested in the intervention. Case recording, program evaluation, accountability reporting, and marketing efforts may also be supplemented by audiovisuals. Drawbacks to recording include intrusiveness or an inhibiting effect, the need to obtain equipment, and the problem of being distracted by the equipment.

The choice of mediums for recording group sessions depends on the facilitator's or agency's objectives and priorities. Videotaping is, of course, the most complete method of recording, but audiotaping can be easier to manage and equally valuable. Before recording group sessions in any format, the facilitator must explain the purpose, ensure confidentiality, and obtain written consent from group (and family) members.

OBSERVING AND
ANALYZING GROUP SESSIONS

An alternative or additional method of documenting the group content and process is to use written observations. Certain aspects of the group as a whole and of each individual can be recorded in each session. A nonparticipatory observer, whose function is explained to the group, can sit to the side and focus solely on this task.

It is difficult to find existing standardized formats for observing group behavior that are relevant to individuals with early-stage dementia. The forms in Figure 5 were adapted from those used for the research described in Chapter 9. The facilitator may choose to modify the forms depending on what he or she wishes to study. General areas of interest may include what the participants talk about and how they interact with one another in the group. For research purposes, Figure 5 needs a significant amount of further development. Quantitative analysis could be designed to measure specifics in a support group, such as the instances of certain nonverbal behaviors. Qualitative or descriptive analysis could capture, for example, what issues were of concern to the group over the 8 weeks, or whether an individual took on a particular role in the group over time.

The forms in Figure 5 can be used in each session—one for the whole group and one for each individual. Each form is first presented blank and then followed by a completed sample to illustrate what the facilitator can expect and how he or she might use the forms.

EVALUATING THE PROGRAM

An evaluation of a new support group is likely to be required and can be helpful to the facilitator and/or the agency sponsoring the group. Feedback may be used to modify and strengthen the intervention, provide reporting data to funding sources and administrative auspices, and document service need and effectiveness as discussed for advocacy, program development, and training purposes. As mentioned previously, the knowledge base in the area of early-stage dementia is just beginning to be built. The perceived benefits, concerns, and suggestions for change discussed by the group will be invaluable to individual providers of support groups, and will advance sophistication in the field of dementia care as a whole.

143

OBSERVATION OF GROUP AS A WHOLE

Session: #   **Date:**

1. **Group topics discussed**
   a. Initiated by facilitator:

   b. Initiated by participants:

2. **Group mood**
   a. Affect:

   b. Relation of mood to themes:

3. Group interactions

a. Turn taking:

b. Interactions among members:

c. Interactions with facilitator:

(continued)

Developing Support Groups for Individuals with Early-Stage Alzheimer's Disease: Planning, Implementation, and Evaluation by Robyn Yale   © 1995 Robyn Yale

Figure 5.   Observation forms adapted from a support group for individuals with early-stage Alzheimer's disease. One form is designed for the whole group and one for each individual.

145

Figure 5. *(continued)*

4. Group facilitation

a. Facilitator's role:

b. Facilitation techniques:

5. Highlights

a. Special problems:

b. Special strengths:

6. Miscellaneous

a. Seating patterns:

b. Absences of members:

c. General impressions/comments:

(continued)

147

Figure 5. *(continued)*

SAMPLE

OBSERVATION OF GROUP AS A WHOLE

Session: # 3   **Date:** *3/12/93*

1. Group topics discussed

a. Initiated by facilitator: *Question–What kinds of things have become more difficult with the onset of dementia? Answer–Everyday things, such as losing something that one just put down, forgetting telephone numbers, forgetting to take medication. Question–How to deal with these? Answer– Trust that things will turn up later, use memory aids, manage stress with physical exercise.*

b. Initiated by participants: *Very difficult to become dependent on others after 60-80 years of being independent.*

2. Group mood

a. Affect: *Frustration, anger, some acceptance, some lighthearted joking*

b. Relation of mood to themes: *Appropriately varied with topics*

3. Group interactions

a. Turn taking: *Question each other about experiences. They don't interrupt.*

b. Interactions among members: *A good deal of camaraderie. Learning from each other (e.g., about the Medic-Alert bracelet, about newspaper clippings on Alzheimer's disease research, exchanging coping techniques)*

c. Interactions with facilitator: *Cooperative, responsive, attentive*

_____

(continued)

*Developing Support Groups for Individuals with Early-Stage
Alzheimer's Disease: Planning, Implementation, and Evaluation*
by Robyn Yale   © 1995 Robyn Yale

149

Figure 5. *(continued)*

4. Group facilitation

a. Facilitator's role: *Offer expertise (e.g., when asked, "Is Alzheimer's disease related to eating certain foods or drinking moderate amounts of alcohol?"), keep meeting focused, provide resource information*

b. Facilitation techniques: *Redirect "tangents," reassure participant who became anxious about wife's whereabouts, check in with quieter group members*

5. Highlights

a. Special problems: *Others forget or sometimes ignore SL's hearing loss.*

b. Special strengths: *Members are able to be jovial as well as serious about their difficulties.*

150

6. Miscellaneous

a. Seating patterns: *Sit in same seats each week (without direction)*

b. Absences of members: *LH–doctor's appointment*

c. General impressions/comments: *Members becoming more self-disclosing. BT told others he finds it "nourishing" to think of the group during the week. Less intervention needed by facilitator today than in first two meetings.*

(continued)

151

Figure 5. *(continued)*

OBSERVATION OF INDIVIDUAL MEMBERS

Name: **Session: #**   **Date:**

1. **Nonverbal behavior**

   a. Expression of emotion:

   b. Facial expressions:

   c. Body language:

   d. Physical behavior:

152

2. Topics

a. Themes raised:

b. Themes responded to (initiated by others):

c. Key phrases:

(continued)

153

Figure 5. *(continued)*

3. Interpersonal behavior

a. Amount and style of relating to others:

b. Amount and style of relating to facilitator:

4. Characteristics

a. Problems in group:

b. Strengths in group:

5. Participation

a. Amount:

b. Type:

c. Communication ability and style:

6. Miscellaneous

a. General impressions:

b. Comments:

(continued)

155

Figure 5. *(continued)*

SAMPLE

OBSERVATION OF INDIVIDUAL MEMBERS

Name: *JD*　　　　**Session:** # *6*　　　　**Date:** *4/3/93*

1. Nonverbal behavior

a. Expression of emotion: *A little tearful when she expressed feelings of sadness and anger.*

b. Facial expressions: *Sad when discussing her children but not throughout meeting.*

c. Body language: *Careful listener. Nods in agreement.*

d. Physical behavior: *Sits very still generally.*

2. Topics

a. Themes raised: *Realizes she needs more assistance with things but doesn't like to be over-protected by family.*

b. Themes responded to (initiated by others): *When KF raised the issue of the uncertainty of the future, she (JD) said, "I just hope for the best, try to do as much for myself as I can."*

c. Key phrases: *"I don't think it's good to hold feelings in–it's better to talk about these things."*

(continued)

157

Figure 5. *(continued)*

3. Interpersonal behavior

a. Amount and style of relating to others: *Smiles and acknowledges others, shows concern but is a bit reserved.*

b. Amount and style of relating to facilitator: *Responds best to very direct questions.*

4. Characteristics

a. Problems in group: *On the quieter side—needs to be drawn out.*

b. Strengths in group: *Always very attentive, thoughtful.*

5. Participation

a. Amount: *Low in comparison to others.*

b. Type: *Always listens. Is focused and on track when she does speak.*

c. Communication ability and style: *A little apprehensive, needs encouragement.*

6. Miscellaneous

a. General impressions: *Says she would like to continue in a group after the 8 weeks—seems to be enjoying it and engaging more than she did initially. Forgot that there would only be two sessions left.*

b. Comments:

Participants can be asked to comment on the group experience during the last session. As suggested in Chapter 5, caregivers can be invited to attend the end of the final meeting, and they can also be asked for their perceptions of the participants' reactions to the group. The facilitator may additionally want to interview each participant and his or her caregiver individually with questionnaires similar to the two in Figure 6. It is important to stress here that these are *not* intended for purposes of assessment or research in which the facilitator's goals are far more complex. For example, attempting to prove "cause and effect" from the intervention or measuring changes in status would necessitate more rigorous investigation. It would also require that the same interview be administered before and after the group experience. The screening and interview forms in Chapter 2 can be adapted for this purpose. Facilitators who have the skills and resources are encouraged to develop and standardize new instruments that can yield quantifiable results more specific to early-stage dementia.

Figure 6 asks for the participants' and caregivers' responses to the program. The facilitator must let the group members know that they are not expected to have retained everything from the sessions—the participants can just comment on their most vivid impressions and feelings.

CONCLUSION

There are many administrative details that must be considered when implementing support groups for individuals with early-stage Alzheimer's disease. Public relations, liability issues, and group fees are among the important areas in which procedures must be developed. The client characteristics, the group experience, and feedback from program participants and their caregivers should all be documented for purposes of accountability, reporting, and evaluation.

EVALUATION OF GROUP BY PARTICIPANTS

Name: **Date:**   **Staff:**

1. What did you enjoy about the group?

2. What did you not like about the group?

3. Is there anything you would change about the group?

4. How has the group been helpful to you?

5. Is there any way in which the group was not helpful to you or made you uncomfortable?

162

6. Do you have any comments about the time, place, or length of meetings?

7. Do you have any comments about the group facilitator?

8. Would you like to continue attending a group? Why or why not?

9. Do you have additional comments?

10. Staff observations and notes (e.g., communication, orientation):

(continued)

Developing Support Groups for Individuals with Early-Stage Alzheimer's Disease: Planning, Implementation, and Evaluation by Robyn Yale © 1995 Robyn Yale

Figure 6. Evaluation questionnaires used to elicit feedback about the support group from the participants and their caregivers.

Figure 6. *(continued)*

EVALUATION OF GROUP BY PARTICIPANTS' CAREGIVERS

Name: **Date:**   **Staff:**

1. What did the participant say about the support group experience?

2. Did the participant mention anything he or she particularly enjoyed about the group?

3. Did the participant mention anything he or she particularly disliked or would like to see changed about the group?

4. How do you think the group was helpful to the participant?

5. Are there any ways that you think the group was not helpful?

6. Did you have any concerns about the participant's response to group participation?

7. Did you notice anything in particular before or after the group meetings in terms of the participant's mood or behavior?

8. Has the participant's support group experience affected you as a caregiver in any way? Describe any effect on how you feel, how you do things, and so forth.

9. Would you like the participant to continue attending a group? Why or why not?

10. Do you have any other comments?

11. Staff observations and notes (e.g., caregiver's view of symptoms, caregiver functioning):

7

INVOLVING CAREGIVERS AND FAMILY MEMBERS

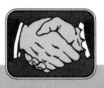

- Family members and the participant selection process
- The role of family members in the support group
- The principle of confidentiality
- Keeping family members informed
- Offering services to family members
- Support groups for the participants' caregivers
- Assessing and addressing the needs of the family
- Follow-up services to the participants and families after the group has concluded

Although the focus of this book has been on people with early-stage Alzheimer's disease as support group participants, it is crucial to incorporate their caregivers and/or family members in the program that is developed. This may mean delineating specific areas of involvement as part of the service to the participants, or it may entail providing concurrent supplemental services to family members. This chapter calls attention to the needs of the caregivers and offers suggestions for meeting those needs.

FAMILY MEMBERS AND THE PARTICIPANT SELECTION PROCESS

The first people to inquire about a support group for individuals with early-stage Alzheimer's disease are often the potential participants' caregivers and family members. Caregivers provide intake information to help the facilitator determine an individual's appropriateness for the group and will also be interviewed as part of the selection process (see Chapter 2).

The guidelines for participant selection in Chapter 1 suggest that the facilitator frankly explain the purpose and nature of the group to the potential participants and their families, and ascertain how they have handled the discussion of the diagnosis of Alzheimer's disease. When asked whether the potential participant ever acknowledges his or her condition, the caregiver's own perspective will usually become evident. For example, do family members say that a doctor once mentioned Alzheimer's disease to the individual but no one ever breathed another word about it? Or, has there been open, periodic communication about the illness in the home? Do family members appear to have insight into the person's illness or to be in denial of it themselves?

One spouse of an individual with dementia said during a telephone screening, "He doesn't know he has Alzheimer's disease, and wouldn't want to go to a group like this—it would be a matter of me deciding it's good for him and pushing him into it." She then stated that her husband gets upset if he thinks something is "wrong with him" and in talking further, agreed with the group leader that he would not be a good candidate for this program.

Each family is unique, and there is no correct way to cope emotionally with Alzheimer's disease. However, it is worth underscoring here that this group is designed for participants who are seeking information and support and should not be offered to anyone under false pretenses. The facilitator might be concerned, for instance, if a caregiver says something like, "My mother refuses to admit she has a memory problem—I want her to come to your group so she'll have to confront it." These types of family dynamics can be very delicate, and a good rule of thumb is for the facilitator to "back off" when encountering them. Services providing support to caregivers could be suggested as an alternative in such a situation.

It is imperative, then, for the facilitator to do his or her best to determine that the goals of the family, the individual, and the group will all be synchronous. Doing so increases the likelihood that issues arising in one arena can be discussed and worked on in the others.

THE ROLE OF FAMILY MEMBERS
IN THE SUPPORT GROUP

Several key points of contact with caregivers have been previously identified. During the process of selecting group participants, family members and caregivers will be interviewed with the participants and also separately to provide important background information. When the group concludes, these family members and caregivers will be asked to help evaluate it by describing the participants' reactions to the experience.

As individuals are enrolled in the group, caregivers can be asked to sign an agreement similar to the one found in Chapter 6. This specifies that they will provide transportation and escort the participant to and from group meetings. A contact person (or two) should also be designated for ongoing communication about the participant's status, any changes in meeting logistics, and in case of an emergency.

Because caregivers will not be participating in the support group, it is helpful to have a method of periodically checking in with them. This might be formally structured through meetings or telephone contact at regular intervals, or occur informally as the need arises. A facilitator must always take care, though, not to talk about the participants in front of them as if they were not there. It is easy to overlook this, especially when a family member urgently approaches the facilitator after a meeting. Out of personal *and* professional courtesy to the participant who may observe this interaction, it is best to schedule a separate time for private discussion.

As mentioned previously, caregivers can be invited to attend part of the last group session. This gives everyone involved a chance to discuss the experience together, to socialize, and to either plan future interaction or say good-bye to one another.

THE PRINCIPLE OF CONFIDENTIALITY

Confidentiality is a basic ground rule in any support group setting and is no less applicable to individuals with early-stage dementia. This can be explained from the outset and clarified as needed. The suggested enrollment agreement (see Chapter 6) lets families know that the facilitator can tell them generally how the participants are doing and what topics emerge in the group, but will not disclose the specifics of what each participant discusses. The importance of this will be demonstrated if, for example, the individuals ventilate about their family members in group sessions. The facilitator may discuss the principle of confidentiality with the group participants when the ground rules are introduced in the first meeting (see Chapter 5). This helps to establish a sense of safety and trust as members come to know one another and share their feelings.

KEEPING FAMILY MEMBERS INFORMED

Although the principle of confidentiality holds true the majority of the time, there are several notable exceptions. Legally speaking, the group facilitator is required to report to appropriate authorities evidence (and in some states, suspicion) of elder abuse, as well as any risk of suicide or potential harm to others. It is important that the facilitator know the reporting laws and procedures in his or her own state. Information is available from the local police, adult protective services, and mental health departments.

If the group leader has concerns about such issues, he or she should speak privately with the participant to further assess the danger. If official reporting does not seem warranted but the facilitator is hesitant to leave the situation unattended, it is best to ask the participant's permission to discuss matters with family members. Caregivers who are so alerted can then take any precautions necessary (see Chapter 6 for further discussion).

The facilitator should also relay any concerns about the group participants' moods or behaviors to their caregivers. Some participants develop symptoms of clinical depression, anxiety, or psychosis in reaction to physical illness or emotional distress. Medical and/or psychiatric evaluation may be needed to determine whether a concurrent condition exists and should be treated, although the underlying dementia cannot be cured.

Finally, if the facilitator becomes concerned that a participant's impairment has progressed to the point where he or she can no longer contribute to the group or benefit from it, the facilitator will need to notify the family as soon as possible. Suggestions for handling this change in status can be found in Chapter 4.

OFFERING SERVICES TO FAMILY MEMBERS

If staffing and resources permit, it is ideal to also offer a group to the caregivers and family members of the participants. Some might find it convenient if this takes place at the same time as the support group for the individuals with Alzheimer's disease, while others might prefer that it be held at a different time so they can have respite from caregiving while the individual is in the group.

Even if there are no facilities to provide a separate service for caregivers, it is likely that they will become acquainted on their own. They may socialize or informally discuss their situations in a nearby location, while the participants meet in the support group. If possible, the facilitator might consider offering a room in the building as a waiting area.

Another alternative to a series of caregiver support group sessions is to offer only one or two meetings for them over the course of the support group for people with Alzheimer's disease. At the very least, intermittent contact with caregivers should be structured through telephone calls or visits. Depending on what route the facilitator chooses, he or she may need to consider the issue of fees in planning any professional services provided to the caregivers.

SUPPORT GROUPS FOR
THE PARTICIPANTS' CAREGIVERS

A support group for caregivers can adopt the structure of most existing caregiver support groups. However, the focus should be unique in that information and support provided are specific to the early stages of dementia. That is, while the long-term nature and implications of the illness are likely to be acknowledged, the emphasis is on understanding and coping with the initial symptoms and resulting adjustments that are typically required.

The research study reported on in Chapter 9 describes the experience of some caregivers who had attended support groups in which issues such as incontinence and nursing home placement were discussed. These particular family members chose not to return to these meetings and stated that it would be more helpful to them to talk about "grieving and going on with life." Individuals in the study who themselves had early-stage Alzheimer's disease also shared this perspective, realizing that they may live in good health and have only mild impairment for an indefinite period of time.

Other program models for caregivers have also been developed. Support groups for people with dementia and their family members together can be offered, with formats including education, discussion, and recreation. Details on these options are beyond the scope of this book because each different format has distinct features and procedures. Ideally, those who have offered these services in the past will make information about them publicly accessible.

ASSESSING AND ADDRESSING THE NEEDS OF THE FAMILY

It is advisable for the group leader to find some way of attending to the caregivers' needs even if he or she is unable to provide them with any formal services. In addition to keeping in touch about the support group as previously discussed, the caregivers' own needs should be assessed at least once and referrals to appropriate community resources offered.

It may be easiest to include this as part of the interviews with the caregivers before and/or after the support group (see Chapter 2). Questions about issues of concern, the physical and mental health of family members, and support systems can point the way to literature (e.g., articles on behavior management, legal planning) that might be helpful and local services (e.g., respite, information and referral) that might be utilized.

FOLLOW-UP SERVICES TO THE PARTICIPANTS AND FAMILIES AFTER THE GROUP HAS CONCLUDED

The extent of follow-up that a facilitator or agency sponsoring a group can provide will depend on the program structure and resources. It may be that all the facilitator can do when the group ends is make referrals to other services in the region. This will be difficult if few services are available in the community. The facilitator should continue to advocate for additional early-stage programs to be developed by others.

Ideally, there should be a *variety* of services for the different levels and transition points within all the stages of Alzheimer's disease. Support groups with different formats, individual and/or family counseling, and care planning or consultation specific to the beginning point in the illness may all be used by those coping with the range of time between mild and moderate impairment. Affordable case management that assists the individuals and their families in obtaining (and accepting) home or day care if those needs arise is also very important.

CONCLUSION

Caregivers and family members of individuals with early-stage Alzheimer's disease have needs that are specific to the beginning point in the illness. Existing caregiver support services have not always made this distinction, and it is important to build it into this new specialized program. Family members are involved at key points in the group for people with Alzheimer's disease, including the participant selection and program evaluation processes. Contact should also be maintained with family members throughout the group session, either informally or through concurrent services provided. The facilitator and/or the agency sponsoring the group must also acknowledge the principle of confidentiality and the need for follow-up services after the group has concluded.

8

USING ROLE PLAYS TO TRAIN GROUP FACILITATORS

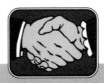

- Setting the stage
- Cast of characters
- Role plays
- Behind the scenes

R ole playing is an excellent training medium for those who will be involved with support groups for individuals with early-stage Alzheimer's disease. Enacting simulated "scenes" from group life, replete with realistic characters and interactions, allows facilitators to preview what the experience will be like and rehearse their own roles within it.

SETTING THE STAGE

It is helpful to anticipate the diversity of personality types, early-stage dementia symptoms, and discussion topics that might occur in group sessions and to practice specific skills and strategies that can be useful across many situations.

Role playing can also be used to educate board and agency staff members (or others involved in sponsoring groups) about the nature, scope, and implications of providing the service. Role playing can also work well as part of a training workshop in which an overview of early-stage Alzheimer's disease is offered. Role play exercises illustrate how individuals at this point in the illness communicate and function, and demonstrate the complexity of issues discussed, techniques, and responses required by the facilitator. This can be useful in finalizing the decision of whether to offer a group and in emphasizing the importance of having qualified coordinators and facilitators to manage it.

Recommended credentials for group facilitators to have and the need for additional specialized training are outlined in Chapter 3. In addition, the art of managing the group process can best be taught initially by someone with a solid clinical background and experience in doing support groups for people with Alzheimer's disease. The training forum might also include the supervisor responsible for the group, as well as colleagues who can offer peer consultation. In addition, involving administrative personnel allows the facilitator to identify and problem-solve potential liability issues, such as handling a medical or behavioral emergency.

The role-play exercises below are drawn from the research study described in Chapter 9, which documents group themes and interactions, and from Chapter 5, which discusses multifaceted group dynamics. The trainer and/or facilitator may want to refer back to these sections in preparation for the role plays.

What follows encompasses some phenomena that are typical of all support groups and some that are unique to groups for this population. Thus, the facilitator must keep in mind that he or she can generalize the experience from other group settings to a support group for people with Alzheimer's disease or conversely, take what is specific to this group and apply it to his or her "generic" knowledge and skills about groups. The facilitator's primary task is always to intervene when necessary in order to keep the environment safe and under control and to enable the group's development and process to be as therapeutic as possible for each participant.

CAST OF CHARACTERS

There are three scenarios below that portray a range of topics, behaviors, events, and personalities that may be typical of the variety found in real groups.

For each situation, the trainer assigns the roles of group facilitator and group members and gives participants their character and scene descriptions. The purpose of the exercises, as described previously, can be reviewed initially, and the "actors" reminded that although they may have fun with this, it is not to be done with ridicule of people with Alzheimer's disease. Actors can then take seats in a circle of chairs, and those who are observing rather than acting should receive an introduction to the scene and its significant aspects.

The role play should run for approximately 15 minutes and be stopped when it seems opportune to do so. Afterward, discussion can be facilitated by the trainer using the questions provided and incorporating any other comments, concerns, and reactions of the participants and observers.

ROLE PLAYS

Role Play #1

1. **Select six volunteers to be in the role play and designate one to be the facilitator and five to be group members.**

2. **Give each actor one of the following written descriptions from which to work:**
    *   You are the leader of a group that has five members. One group member brings up her struggle to accept the idea that she needs help in the home. Each of the other members has a different reaction to this. You must delicately facilitate this discussion so that all points of view and coping styles are acknowledged and respected, while also sharing your own perspective on the issue.

- You are a group member who lives alone and has been advised by your family to hire in-home help. You are struggling with your feelings about this and discussing the pros and cons to make a decision.
- You are a group member who responds to another member that you, too, at first resisted getting in-home help but finally came to terms with it and now have someone. You explain how you feel about it and whether it has been a good decision for you. You might speak just a bit slowly and forgetfully so that your impairment is noticeable, but it is still possible to clearly discuss this issue.
- You are a group member who, although trying to be supportive, is actually giving advice based on your own denial. That is, in a discussion about getting in-home help you tend to minimize your own impairments and be overly optimistic about doing well without any help indefinitely, so you figure others can, too.
- You are a group member who finds the whole discussion of needing in-home help overwhelming and gets tearful or upset while sharing your feelings on the subject.
- You are a group member who, in a discussion about needing in-home help, offers positive support, particularly to the person struggling with a decision about this and to the person who becomes upset. Occasionally, you have trouble finding a word or two, but this is not too disruptive—you are able to just talk through it.

3. **Instruct the players to enact the following scene:**
   The group is talking about the different ways in which life has changed as a result of having Alzheimer's dis-

ease, and one participant is struggling with accepting the need for help in the home. Each participant has a different perspective on this issue, and the group leader carefully facilitates the discussion.

4. **Give the audience the following questions as a basis for discussion after the exercise:**
   - What do you see as the biggest challenge for the facilitator in this group session?
   - Is there anything that surprises you about what the group members say and how they interact with one another?
   - Imagine yourself as the group leader in this situation. Would you feel confident, or do you have concerns about how you would handle things that you would like to discuss?

5. **Note to trainer**
   The issue in this role play is one of the most difficult and poignant for individuals with Alzheimer's disease—that of facing increasing dependency and resulting changes in lifestyle. Each person faces this in his or her own way and time, and group members can support one another in accepting it but cannot force the process. It is always important for the facilitator to monitor this and to point out that everyone has a unique response and the right to not be judged or pressured by others.

   The facilitator must try to balance honest acknowledgment of potential disease progression with reinforcement for the participants' current high levels of functioning. It is likely that group members will help to create this balance because they are experiencing the reality of both aspects.

Finally, this role play illustrates some of the challenges and rewards of group work with individuals who have Alzheimer's disease. Even those in the early stages are at different points in the disease process and in the process of accepting their limitations. Denial and strong emotional reactions are possible within the group, but there are also likely to be shared coping strengths. Cognitive impairment will occur in group sessions, but participants can still be competent in expressing themselves. And, the facilitator's key roles here, as in other groups, include providing information, maintaining mutual respect for each participant's boundaries, and monitoring the distinction between appropriate problem solving and intrusive advice giving.

Role Play #2

1. **Select five volunteers to be in the role play and designate one to be the facilitator and four to be group members.**

2. **Give each actor one of the following written descriptions from which to work:**
   - You are the group facilitator with four group members who are asking you questions about Alzheimer's disease. The discussion leads to the issue of driving, and everyone has a different reaction and opinion on the subject.
   - You are a group member who starts things off with questions about Alzheimer's disease, such as "How do they know I have Alzheimer's?", "What does the word 'Alzheimer's' mean?", and "What kinds of tests do they do to diagnose it?"

When the issue of driving comes up you ask something like, "How does the 'driving board' know to come after a person's license? What if you can still drive perfectly well?"

Feel free to add any other questions or comments that may occur to you in the discussion.

- You are a group member who is very angry because you just had your driver's license revoked. You do not understand what driving has to do with Alzheimer's disease. You feel your family and your doctor are against you on this one, and you do not know what to do about it all.

- You are a group member who knows a lot about Alzheimer's disease and can answer some of the questions asked by others. You are able to stay calm and be supportive while saying things like, "Having Alzheimer's can make it harder to concentrate while driving," or "They give you a driving test to see if you can still drive safely," and even, "After all, none of us wants to cause an accident, do we?"

- You are a group member who has more cognitive impairment, and this shows itself as you go off on a tangent. When the discussion turns to driving, you bring up a story about a car you used to own and ramble on a bit, off the subject of losing a driver's license. At other points in the discussion, you might start to say something and lose your train of thought once or twice.

3. **Instruct the players to enact the following scene:**
The group is discussing what Alzheimer's disease is and the issue of driving comes up. This raises further questions and members share their concerns and experiences.

4. **Give the audience the following questions as a basis for discussion after the exercise:**
   - How well do you think the facilitator answered the group members' questions about Alzheimer's disease? Would this be difficult for you to do?
   - Would you try anything different to handle the person who has more cognitive impairment?
   - What might the person who is angry and the person who goes off on a tangent have in common?

5. **Note to trainer**
   Both the angry group member and the person reminiscing about a favorite old car are probably dealing with issues of grief and loss. It can be helpful for the facilitator to identify and validate the feelings that may occur in reaction to the current loss of a driver's license.

   Although it is difficult to be asked questions about Alzheimer's disease, remember that members have come to the group for such information and typically have not had much opportunity to discuss it before. Be sure you know the facts about the illness yourself as well as any relevant resources. And in this case, be prepared to explain the law that exists in your region about driving and dementia.

   This scenario has a smaller group size, which can be challenging. In small groups each person is very apparent and all are likely to participate. Although six to eight is an ideal number of participants, there may be occasional absences, drops in attendance, or times of low enrollment. However, this is fine, as four members certainly constitute a group.

   It is wonderful when group members can educate and calm one another, as happened here. As far as the tangential member, he or she can be brought back to the discussion with gentle reminding of the relevance of their anecdote to the driving issue. This scenario also demonstrates a participant who may need to be monitored or reevaluated to be sure he or she does not have too much cognitive impairment to be in the group.

Role Play #3

1. Select seven volunteers to be in the role play and designate one to be the facilitator and six to be group members.

2. Give each actor one of the following written descriptions from which to work:
    *   You are the facilitator of a group with six members. There is one session left after today and then the group ends. You review generally what the meetings have been like and ask for feedback from the participants about what they have liked or disliked about the program. You are able to share with the group that you feel sad to say good-bye to them and other similar feelings. You also help them say good-bye to one another and to make plans for getting support when the group is no longer meeting.
    *   You are a group member who feels the group has become like family and friends to you. As the discussion focuses on the group ending next week, you express your gratitude to particular participants and the group as a whole for the support and help you have received.
    *   You are a group member who is uncomfortable with discussing that the group will end next week,

so you keep changing the subject or cutting off other people who are expressing emotion about this.

• You are a group member who is very afraid of the group ending next week because you fear what will happen if the disease gets worse for you. You are able to be honest and reach out to others about this.

• You are a group member who is optimistic about the future and is able to reassure others who are anxious about the group ending next week. You remind your peers about some of the coping skills that have been discussed in the group (humor, activity, etc.).

• You are a group member who is attentive but not participating much in the discussion about the group ending next week. When you do speak a few times, you do so quietly and not very clearly due to your difficulty with speech. You make it obvious, though, that you are able to understand the conversation.

• You are a group member who shares with the group that you plan to start going to a day center after this group ends. You explain what the center is like and why you have decided to go.

3. **Instruct the players to enact the following scene:**

    The group will be ending after next week's session. Members are discussing what the experience has been like and planning for support and connection in the future. Different issues and feelings are coming up for the participants, as well as for the facilitator.

4. **Give the audience the following questions as a basis for discussion after the exercise:**

   - What do you think are the pros and cons of having a time-limited group with an endpoint like this versus an open-ended group where individual members leave the group at different times?

   - How is this group session the same as or different from others you have facilitated?

   - What do you think are some of the benefits this group has had for its participants?

5. **Note to trainer**

   Termination is inevitable with groups, but is rarely easy. Starting the termination process at least two sessions in advance prepares everyone (including the group leader) for this upcoming transition. Giving the subject plenty of time and attention helps group members work through their feelings about ending the experience and provides the facilitator with feedback by which to evaluate the program.

   It is important to give each participant a chance to acknowledge his or her perspective on the group ending, and some may need assistance to articulate this, such as the participant who cut off discussion in the above example. It can be instructive to explicitly ask what was helpful and not helpful about the group, how members would like to say good-bye to one another, and specifically how they plan to continue finding support on an ongoing basis.

   As in any group setting, termination of the support group for individuals with Alzheimer's disease may evoke powerful emotional reactions related to feelings of loss. However, it can also be a prime opportunity for emphasizing and consolidating what has been gained from the group experience. Again, each person will have his or her unique way of coping with this developmental step.

The facilitator must be appropriate about his or her own reactions to termination. It is okay to share relevant feelings but not to need emotional support or assistance from group members. Outside supervision or therapy is the best way to have one's own issues addressed and attended to.

BEHIND THE SCENES

The three role plays above are only a starting point in the training needed to be the facilitator of a support group for individuals with Alzheimer's disease. Of course, it is not possible to predetermine how group sessions will go or how a person might respond as a group leader in every situation that occurs. Rather, it is hoped that these exercises provide a preview of the depth of issues, feelings, and dynamics that are possible in a group setting with this population.

However, these vivid examples should not cause "stage fright." Although they convey an intensity and complexity the facilitator may find intimidating, role playing is a medium for orientation and ongoing learning, trial and error, and clinical guidance. No one could be expected to know how to handle all of these behaviors and situations without some preparation, instruction, and ultimately, experience.

CONCLUSION

In most instances, there is no right way to respond. A good facilitator uses a combination of intuition and professional judgment, feeling his or her way along as the scenario unfolds. The purpose of these exercises is to help the facilitator delineate and ground his or her own approach, refine skills, and clarify the rules and roles as a group leader. Developing and practicing ahead of time fortifies the facilitator's repertoire and increases the confidence to trust and rely on his or her own skills.

The learning process does not stop here. It should be viewed as ongoing as the facilitator goes from this theatrical milieu to the milieu of an actual support group, which in turn mirrors what goes on in "real life." If the facilitator feels that more practice is needed, other exercises can be created using events that he or she would like to practice or problem-solve before they actually happen. An example of this might be the integration of a new member into the group, or the response of the group when one participant needs to leave the group before the 8-week session is over. Once a group begins, role playing can continue to be used as a learning tool for the facilitator by taking what happens in actual group sessions to peer consultation and supervision meetings for feedback from his or her colleagues.

9

RESEARCH STUDY ON SUPPORT GROUPS FOR INDIVIDUALS WITH EARLY DEMENTIA

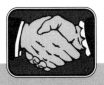

- Research questions
- Procedures
- The sample
- The intervention
- Data collection and analysis
- Results
- Discussion

SUPPORT GROUPS
FOR PATIENTS NEWLY DIAGNOSED
WITH EARLY-STAGE ALZHEIMER'S DISEASE:
HOW PATIENTS MANAGE THEIR CONCERNS

This study was funded by a Pilot Research Grant from the National Alzheimer's Association and conducted in 1992 at University of California, San Francisco, by: Joseph Barbaccia, M.D., Principal Investigator; Linda Mitteness, Ph.D., Coprincipal Investigator; Robyn Yale, L.C.S.W., Project Director; and Catherine Lee, M.A., Research Assistant.

RESEARCH QUESTIONS

"I felt really <u>good</u> doing something for myself...I've gotten so much out of it. It may be helpful for my wife too...she knows I'm trying...I'm not a quitter!"

This study explored how patients with early dementia respond to a professionally led peer support group focused on understanding and coping with Alzheimer's disease. Research questions included the following:

1. Can patients with early dementia express their concerns about Alzheimer's disease in a support group?
2. Will these concerns change after the intervention and several months later?

195

3. Will the support group affect the emotional health and social functioning of these patients?
4. Will the patients' participation in a support group affect the level of burden in their caregivers?

PROCEDURES

Fifteen patients with early-stage Alzheimer's disease and their caregivers were assigned to either treatment or control conditions. The treatment consisted of eight weekly group meetings for the patients only, focused on education and support around the illness. Group sessions were observed, documented, and analyzed. The "controls" received only usual care (in the settings from which they were referred) during this period and were offered a patient support group when data collection was completed. All the patients and their caregivers were interviewed at three points in time: before and after the intervention, and an average of 2 months later. The third interview with all study participants concluded with an offer of general consultation and referral to appropriate community resources.

THE SAMPLE

Because the manifestation and course of Alzheimer's disease differs for each patient, the distinction of "newly diagnosed" did not turn out to be a useful one. The target population was redefined as "early stage," as determined by mild impairment on cognitive testing and interview responses. A score of 18–24 on Folstein's Mini-Mental Status Exam[1] was used as one selection criterion.

---

[1]Folstein, M.F., Folstein, S., & McHugh, P.R. (1975). Mini-mental state: A practical method for grading the cognitive state of patients for the clinician. *Journal of Psychiatric Research, 12,* 189–198.

Only patients who had been told that they probably had Alzheimer's disease (by a physician and/or family member), at least occasionally acknowledged their memory loss, could potentially communicate their feelings and experiences about the illness, and were willing and able to give informed consent could participate in the study. All the patients had a documented diagnosis of probable or possible Alzheimer's disease most recently evaluated within the previous approximate 2 years, and three had additional dementia-related diagnoses. None had other significant medical or psychiatric conditions. Each patient had a family caregiver who was willing to be interviewed and with whom contact occurred at least several times a week.

Participants were recruited through media coverage as well as referrals from the many Alzheimer's service providers in the San Francisco Bay Area. Although 76 inquiries were received initially, only 15 patients were subsequently enrolled. Study inclusion criteria were not met in most instances. For example, approximately one third of those who were interested in the support group were inquiring on behalf of a patient whose cognitive impairment was too advanced to participate and/or who was likely to have behavioral or social difficulties in the group. More than one fifth of the calls related to patients who had either not been told—or were told but denied—their diagnosis. In these instances, in which caregivers wanted patients to participate so they would "face and accept" their condition, it was explained that this was not the project's intent.

Contact with the project was initiated in some cases by the patients themselves, who had learned of the study through newspaper articles. In all cases, caregivers provided historical information during a telephone screening and intake process. Staff then spoke briefly to the patient on the telephone to explain the study, assess initial comprehension and interest, and seek permission to set up an enrollment interview. Consent was secured for the patient's medical records to be reviewed by the principal investigator. Interviews with those eligible were held by two staff members, who met with each patient and caregiver jointly and then separately in the home or research office.

Patients were assigned to either a treatment or control group based on such factors as transportation and scheduling constraints, rather than by their characteristics or abilities. Study participants were diverse in age, gender, ethnicity, and family constellation. A final sample of 13 completed the project: 7 in the support group and 6 in the control group.

THE INTERVENTION

The intervention consisted of eight weekly support group sessions that each lasted 1½ hours. The group was facilitated by the project director, a licensed clinical social worker, who had previously developed a training manual for leaders of patient support groups.

A circle of chairs "set the stage" for the meetings. The facilitator reviewed the purpose and ground rules at the start of each session, providing structure and direction while encouraging group decision making and monitoring participation. Discussion was kept as focused and uncomplicated as possible by raising one issue at a time and continually clarifying and reframing main points. Topics were suggested by the facilitator but increasingly initiated by the patients over time. Examples of themes, such as adapting to cognitive loss and changes in family relationships, are elaborated further in this chapter.

Patients were amazingly able to raise difficult issues, share their feelings, "educate" one another, and commit themselves to the project goals. Although interaction between members was fostered, each patient's style and boundaries were also respected. For example, patients in periodic denial were not forcefully confronted. Overall, because participants were carefully screened before enrollment and welcomed the opportunity to discuss the illness, the need for the facilitator to intervene was less than had been anticipated.

Techniques used by the facilitator accommodated the patients' cognitive impairments. For example, the forgetfulness that occurred within the group was attributed to the disease process, identified as common among group members, and compared to problems occurring outside of the group as well (e.g., *"What do you do in other situations when you have trouble finding a word?"*). Patients having difficulty expressing themselves were asked whether they wanted assistance, and, if so, the facilitator restated, interpreted, and checked the accuracy of what was intuited. The patients' abilities as well as their limitations were acknowledged (e.g., *"You seem able to communicate well in the group—what can help you do that when stressful situations come up elsewhere?"*).

Patients were brought to the meetings and picked up by their caregivers, who often congregated and chatted informally while waiting. The caregivers attended the last session to discuss the group with the patients and staff, exchange names and telephone numbers, and say goodbye to one another.

DATA COLLECTION AND ANALYSIS

Study data consisted of interviews, documentation of support group sessions, and evaluation of the group experience.

1. Three interviews were conducted separately with all
    the patients and caregivers. The first was conducted
    at enrollment (T1), the second after the 8-week sup-
    port group period (T2), and the third an average of 2
    months later (T3). It was not possible to unearth any
    existing measurement tools that assessed status or
    pinpointed concerns specific to early-stage Alzheim-
    er's disease. Therefore, validated instruments were
    supplemented by clinical interviews constructed by
    the research team.

    The patients were assessed at all three points in
    time on Folstein's Mini-Mental Status Exam and the
    Global Deterioration Scale[2] to determine the level of
    cognitive impairment, and on the Hamilton Rating
    Scale for Depression.[3] A semi-structured question-
    naire (based on the domains of the Linn Social Dys-
    function Rating Scale[4]) was administered, which cov-
    ered mood, changes in social relationships and activity
    level, and the patients' perceptions of, adjustments to,
    and concerns about their condition.

    Caregivers were administered scales of depres-
    sion and burden using a subset of the Stress and Cop-
    ing Interview developed by Pearlin, Mullan, Semple,
    and Skaff.[5] Other interview questions developed by

    [2]Reisberg, B., Ferris, S.H., de Leon, M.J., & Crook, T. (1982). The
Global Deterioration Scale for assessment of primary dementia. *American Journal of Psychiatry, 139,* 1136–1139.

    [3]Hamilton, M. (1960). A Rating Scale for Depression. *Journal of
Neurology, Neurosurgery, and Psychiatry, 23,* 56–62.

    [4]Linn, M.W., Sculthorpe, W.B., Evje, M., Slater, P.H., & Goodman,
S.P. (1969). A Social Dysfunction Rating Scale. *Journal of Psychiatric Research, 6,* 299–306.

    [5]Pearlin, L.I., Mullan, J.T., Semple, S.J., & Skaff, M.M. (1990).
Caregiving and the stress process: An overview of concepts and their
measures. *The Gerontologist, 30*(5), 583–591.

the research team covered the caregivers' perceptions of the patients' reactions to the illness, and the impact of the illness on the patients' and families' lives.

2. Support group sessions were observed by a trained research assistant and audiotaped to capture themes and interactions. A specific format was developed to document the process of the group as a whole and record each participant's affect, behavior, and nonverbal communication at every meeting. Areas covered included topics initiated by patients, emotions expressed, levels of participation, and interpersonal styles.

3. Patients who were in the support group were asked to evaluate the group at T2. Caregivers of these participants were asked for their impressions of the patients' responses to the group experience at T2 and T3.

Study data were analyzed by the coprincipal investigator using both quantitative and qualitative techniques. Examination of the established assessment scales followed the model of a repeated measures analysis of variance. As a result of the small sample size, only large differences between treatment and control groups were found to be significant. Results of these statistical analyses need to be interpreted with caution in light of the small sample size and are, therefore, supplemented with a focus on the specific responses of patients and caregivers.

Interviews and support group observations were subjected to limited (primarily nonparametric) statistical analyses and were categorized using standard qualitative methods. Coding strategies were first developed by the whole research team, and, thus, interobserver reliability was established before any responses were coded. A sequential data analysis model was then used, looking first for similarities and patterns within groups, then for changes over time, and finally for differences between groups.

RESULTS

Interviews with Patients with Early-Stage Alzheimer's Disease and Their Caregivers

Patients' Concerns

The patients were willing and able to discuss the impact of memory loss and their feelings about it in interviews. The patients described an awareness of inabilities to do things they had always done and concerns about problems they might eventually develop. Most were able to identify specific areas of difficulty. For example, one knew that, *"Remembering words is the problem....If I try to give an answer immediately I can't do it—I need time."* Another patient remarked, *"I get frustrated when I'm with too many people at once—I can't get the fun they are having and feel very bad about that."*

Patients had varying degrees of acceptance of the changes in their lives. At one end of the spectrum was the person who explained, *"I look at it philosophically. Everyone's going to die and doesn't know how it will happen... if I didn't have Alzheimer's disease it might be something else."* Another expressed a different viewpoint, *"I feel angry—why me¿!! I can't do the things I used to do."* When asked whether they worry about anything in particular, one patient admitted, *"I don't think I'll ever go back to how I was and it scares me. I wish I could do something about it."*

The experiences of being interviewed *and* attending a support group seemed to make the patients feel understood and therefore able to *"do something about it."* For example, one concluded the first interview on a note of hope and determination, exclaiming, *"I feel better already—I feel I can do this!"*

The patients in the support group were found to be more likely to discuss problems related to their illness than were the controls. Patients in the support group were also more likely than the controls to acknowledge that their diagnosis was Alzheimer's disease when asked at the second interview and were significantly more open about Alzheimer's disease with their caregivers at this point in time than they had been initially. In contrast, only one patient in the control group had discussed and made plans regarding the illness at the time of the second interview. By the third interview, several patients who had been in the support group were seeking information about other dementia-related services, such as day programs and individual therapy specific to Alzheimer's disease.

Caregivers' Perceptions of Patients' Concerns

Caregivers described major changes in patients' social lives, work lives, relationships, and identities: *"He was always an active scientist and intellectual and is no longer capable of that. An entire reassessment of himself and his future was necessary."* Many previous activities had been affected by the illness: *"Socializing has decreased...he never wants to go out. He feels self-conscious, that he won't know how to interact with friends anymore."*

Caregivers sensed that patients had mixed feelings about the explanation for their symptoms. One noted some positive aspects: *"Sometimes he feels the loss; yet, there's also relief [about the diagnosis] because things have been effortful for years without knowing why. He's now happier, more relaxed, and more emotionally avail-*

able." Another commented on her relative's loneliness: *"She'd like to do more [socially] but she's unsure of herself—she's scared that she won't be able to make herself understood."*

Several caregivers mentioned that they had discussed worries about the future with the patients as increasing cognitive and functional impairment became more apparent: *"He's appropriately concerned—he worries what will happen if he becomes unable to talk."* Some agreed together on preferences for long-term care arrangements: *"He's concerned about me [wife] working too hard.... He asked me to promise that I would place him in a nursing home if he later becomes a burden for me."*

Caregivers' Concerns

When asked about any changes that were newly troublesome for them, caregivers identified shifting roles and relationships with patients: *"I'm now the only breadwinner and caretaker...ours was a very equitable relationship, we always made joint decisions after lengthy discussion—I miss this interaction."* Loss of intimacy was mentioned by some of the caregivers as well: *"There have been sexual changes. Sex is less frequent and she is fearful of it."*

Caregivers related other stresses, such as isolation, the need for respite, and lack of family consensus around care needs. The patients' dependency and resistance were also reported as difficult at times. One example was having to talk to the person differently: *"I have lots of frustration around the constant need for clarification and repetition—I feel angry and then feel bad about that."* Another commented, *"She is more oppositional when you try to help her with things, which exasperates me."*

A few of the caregivers who had themselves attended community support groups felt that their needs were different from those of individuals caring for patients with later-stage Alzheimer's disease. One caregiver stated strongly that none of the existing literature or services she had encountered addressed early-stage Alzheimer's disease in terms of *"constructing a life, grieving, and going on rather than just dealing with the long-term picture."*

Assessment of Patients and Caregivers

Patient Status

Generally, assessment data did not indicate statistically significant differences between those patients who were in a support group and those who were not. However, it is difficult to know whether this speaks to the effect of the intervention, the imprecision of existing measurement tools, the impact of the small sample size on statistical analyses, or a combination of these and other factors. This is one reason that the study was set up with a process-oriented emphasis, focusing less on outcomes and more on the patients' abilities and responses in the support group. For the sake of completion, data on the cognitive, emotional, and social functioning of patients are, however, reported below and should be interpreted with caution, as previously stated.

Patients in both treatment and control groups had mean scores representing mild cognitive impairment on Folstein's Mini-Mental Status Exam and the Global Deterioration Scale. All remained within this range over time, although there was some individual decline within each group. Improvement had not been expected among support group participants, given that all patients with Alzheimer's disease decline cognitively at an unpredictable but continuous rate.

None of the individual or mean scores for either group, at any of the measurement times, reached significance for clinical depression as measured by the Hamilton

Rating Scale for Depression. The impact of group participation on the patients' emotional health was difficult to evaluate, however, particularly because several were reacting to other crises (e.g., death of friends or relatives) at T2. Overall, the patients in the support group were neither significantly more distressed, worried, or sad (i.e., after learning more about the effects of Alzheimer's disease or after the end of their group experience), nor were they significantly more cheerful, happy, or calm (i.e., after sharing experiences with others and knowing they were not alone). The patients stated that their self-esteem was higher as a result of support group participation and reported such mood-related benefits as, *"It took away the embarrassment. It made me feel more hopeful, hearing how people cope, knowing you have plenty of options."*

There were no significant changes over time in either group's social functioning in terms of leisure activity level, paid or volunteer work, or relationships. Friends and family were among the topics discussed within support group sessions, though. For example, one patient who was sad that he rarely saw his friends since the onset of Alzheimer's disease decided to set up special one-to-one visits with them, after coming to understand that socializing with several people at once increased his confusion.

The patients in the support group reported enjoying each other and described a sense of belonging, but did not consider the group to be a social activity. Most of these patients recalled and wanted to continue the group experience at the time of third interview, while most of the control patients were still feeling isolated and had not done much to address the illness.

Caregiver Status
Caregivers in treatment and control groups were assessed as relatively equal in terms of their own emotional status,

reporting moderate levels of anger expressed, anxiety, depression, and general overload. Scores on these scales were not significantly different between groups nor did they change significantly over time. However, it was difficult to determine the effect patient support group participation had on caregiver burden, particularly because several caregivers reported dealing with other crises (e.g., moving) at T2. Although one could speculate that caregiver stress might be reduced if the patients' well-being improved, this is quite difficult to quantify and measure.

Caregivers did describe the patients' support group experience as helpful to their relatives as well as to themselves. When asked at T2 whether there had been any effect on how they felt or the way they did things, one caregiver stated, *"I used to feel guilty [because I had my own activities]...I felt good that my husband was participating in something that he saw as his. It helped me to know that he was trying to deal with the illness; he had a place he could talk to others."* Several caregivers mentioned having learned about other available services, *"My husband said one group member did volunteer work in an Alzheimer['s disease] day program—he was interested in that kind of [social/recreational] opportunity. Do you have information on this?"* For the daughter of one participant, the group provided a break from caregiving responsibilities. And another caregiver explained the benefit of the group for the whole family, *"My mother is more confident and less anxious about her condition. The group brought things into the open, which was a great relief. Now there's less mystery around discussing the disease at home."* Finally, one caregiver felt less isolated after her relative's experience: *"Even though the group wasn't for me it helped to meet other patients and caregivers—most people don't know what we're going through; any connections or understanding I get helps."*

Support Group Content and Process

Content of Patients' Concerns in Group

The patients in the support group had the motivation and capacity to articulate their questions, experiences, emotions, and coping strategies. Topics ranged widely and commonalities among group members emerged immediately. For example, one person discovered in the first meeting that he was not the only one who had had his driving privileges revoked. All of the others had also dealt with this. Although some had resigned to accept it, a few had attempted to appeal the action. Several knew the state law regarding dementia and driving and were able to explain it to those less familiar with it. The patients also raised their awareness of the stereotyped image of a person with Alzheimer's disease and expressed hope that they could challenge the stigma of "becoming an imbecile" by participating in this research project. The patients balanced humor and optimism about their current wellness with acknowledging everyday frustrations and the uncertainty of the future. Major themes are summarized in the following list to illustrate the nature and depth of discussion:

- *Diagnosis of Alzheimer's disease*—How Alzheimer's disease is diagnosed and distinguished from normal memory loss, what it was like to experience diagnostic testing (e.g., felt like a child, felt "dumb" going through it) and to realize the extent of one's impairments in this setting, general questions about the cause and course of the disease

- *Stigma*—Awareness that patients with Alzheimer's disease are often perceived as "6 feet under already," erroneous assumptions that patients will be more physically and mentally incapacitated than they are, others often do things for patients that they can do themselves

208

- *Changes in lifestyle and/or abilities*—Adjusting to having one's career end prematurely; difficulty with speaking, writing, or adding numbers; getting lost; using coping strategies (e.g., "word substitution")
- *Driving*—Reasons for and reactions to having driving privileges revoked, legal and safety concerns around dementia and driving, loss of independence that results from giving up license
- *Dependency*—Getting used to needing assistance from others (e.g., with transportation), the struggle to accept help but function as independently as possible, changes in established marital roles (e.g., wife newly managing all finances)
- *Family*—Concern that family members do not understand that certain behaviors are due to the illness (e.g., "I wish my wife would see that I don't do these things on purpose. I'm doing my best—sometimes, she yells at me"), patients cognizant of the strain on family members who must repeat themselves and try various ways to communicate (e.g., "It's not that I'm ignoring her"), patients' love for their family members and deep appreciation for the care provided to them
- *Friends*—The loss that is felt when friends "disappear" because they can no longer relate to patients; the need to educate friends who are fearful or misinformed about Alzheimer's disease and to structure comfortable visits; the difficulty when friends expect patients to be worse than they are, or conversely, when friends minimize what patients are going through (in an effort to be supportive)
- *Communication*—Becomes easier when things are slowed down and simplified, and conversely is more difficult with more people and stimuli; patients can let others know what works and what does not in this re-

gard; the need for patients to expect less from themselves in this area

- *Alzheimer's disease*—Interest in current research being done (e.g., medications), great frustration that research has not yet produced a cure for Alzheimer's disease, satisfaction that they were offering new information and potentially helping others through participation in this study
- *Wellness and optimism*—The patients' realization that they may live for many years, with an unpredictable rate of disease progression; the idea of not dwelling on the future, but rather taking it "a day at a time"; the importance of pleasurable activities and support systems
- *Preparing for the future*—The necessity of advance legal planning, local resources available and services patients (and their families) have utilized, the importance of discussing the illness with family and friends
- *The group*—The benefit of having the group so that people can learn and talk about Alzheimer's disease, the hope that other groups will be developed for other patients with Alzheimer's disease, reviewing and ending this group experience

Observations of Patients' Interactions in Group

The patients became cohesive from the start of meetings and were very engaging, open, and supportive with one another. They assisted each other in specific subject areas as well as with such incidents as helping a member who was more frail into her seat or suggesting that an individual with hearing loss use a sign saying "LOUDER, PLEASE" as needed.

Group members treated each other with tolerance and kindness, particularly in regard to difficulty with either cognitive or emotional expression. They became increasingly relaxed and self-disclosing over time. Conversation was sustained and all of the patients participated, although as might be expected, some were more verbal than others. The patients were cooperative with the facilitator and needed less direction after the first few sessions. Although they were willing to discuss difficult issues and feelings, they also respected one another's limits. For instance, one patient's initial denial regarding her impairments eventually subsided after being gently approached by others (e.g., *"I see, maybe you don't have the same problems as us . . . but why are you coming here, then?"*).

Affect was appropriately responsive and varied—at some times serious, pensive, and realistic; at other times hopeful and upbeat. Nonverbal behavior usually reflected interest, as in leaning forward or looking at each other when speaking. Humor and good-natured banter occurred often, as illustrated by comments like, *"We're getting so comfortable here, soon we'll be borrowing money from each other!"* and *"Oh sure, you'll remember what you were about to say—I've heard that one before!"*

Although the ability of patients with Alzheimer's disease to retain group support has been questioned, there were obvious indications that participants recalled and valued the experience. For example, they appeared glad to see each other, and many greeted one another by name each week. Interestingly, most patients also chose to sit in the same seat for every meeting, and absences of members were always noticed. In addition, anecdotes relevant to previous sessions were often shared (e.g., *"I felt better after we talked about driving and I held on to this all week to tell you: my wife had trouble parking the car one day— I had to do it for her!"*).

Overall, group members helped each other explore and come to terms with what they were facing, as illustrated by the following:

1. **Examples of Patients Sharing Understanding and Knowledge About Alzheimer's Disease**
   - *"It's important that we all stay healthy. Many patients with Alzheimer's disease die of other illnesses, like pneumonia."*
   - *"The reason you have trouble writing [like I do] is because the brain cells aren't connecting to your hand when you need them to."*
   - *"I'm like you, when I'm pressured, electric currents go every which way and I lose it completely. In fact, that's what happened in the [diagnostic testing], and they concluded I had Alzheimer's disease."*
   - *"What is this experimental medication you're on? Can I get in on that research too?"*
   - *"I volunteer at a day center for patients with Alzheimer's disease. I enjoy helping with the meals and activities they have."*
   - *"If your sister doesn't understand you, she could go to a support group—they have them for what they now call 'caregivers.'"*

2. **Examples of Sharing Feelings and Experiences with One Another**
   - *"Am I the only one who hates the word Alzheimer's?"*
   - *"Do you have this problem, too [reading, speaking, etc.]?"*
   - *"I'm getting used to the idea that I might get worse. I didn't accept it before, but I'm starting to see some changes. Psychologically it seems useful to come to terms with this. What do others of you think?"*

212

- *"I'm not sure what to say—I've lost the thought"...
  [another patient] "That's okay—that happens to
  me a lot!"*

3. **Examples of Sharing Perspectives on the Illness**
   - *"When you think about the people who were in the
     Oakland hills fire or the L.A. riots you have to ad-
     mit that we're better off than they are—things
     could be worse."*
   - *"It's been a big adjustment and loss not being able
     to work anymore. But it's important to find new
     things to do and enjoy—if you just give up, it's like
     wanting to die. Your mood can help you get used to
     the changes."*
   - *"Now I realize I do have a problem, but I'm not
     alone. It's not the end of the world. You've found a
     way to go on with your lives."*

**Patients' and Caregivers'
Responses to the Patients' Group Experience**

Patients' Evaluation of the Group

The patients generally had positive responses to the
group experience and most could identify specific topics
they found helpful to discuss. Only one member who
was in a convalescent facility after knee surgery and was
more confused than other patients at T2, had difficulty
remembering her group experience. Patients described
what they enjoyed about the group during the second interview:

- *"It's okay to share feelings—I don't talk much usually.
  I hold inside too much. This helped me try to make my
  wife understand me."*

213

- *"I liked not being embarrassed to speak up about things I couldn't [describe] before. And everybody understood...had the same ideas and feelings."*
- *"It helped me a lot to organize my thoughts. The feeling of the group was very positive."*

The patients had a sense of altruism and accomplishment about attending the group:

- *"I felt good about myself for talking [and] making new friends."*
- *"I felt good that maybe I was able to help others, too...I pushed the fact that everyone should go to an attorney for advice."*

The patients stated that they felt comfortable with and close to the other group members:

- *"I felt decent and supported. I won't be going to movies with them, but it was important to do what we did: Come in, speak with people, and go out. It never occurred to me to do something with them [other than be in group], yet there was not one negative idea."*
- *"My wife and I developed a relationship with Mr. H. and his wife—they are very fine people. His diagnosis was just this past January, while mine was several years ago!"*

None of the patients mentioned anything that made them uncomfortable, and all expressed a desire to continue in a group. They were surprised and frustrated by the lack of similar services available in the region. One put it this way: *"My wife is always going to caregiver groups—this one was needed for us!"*

Caregivers' Perceptions of Patients' Group Experience

The caregivers reported that patients generally seemed excited each week about the upcoming meeting and made positive comments about the group. One caregiver said that her husband would not discuss the content of the meetings with her because, he explained, what went on in them was confidential. Most caregivers, however, stated that the patients talked about specific topics discussed, liked other group members, and had feelings of relief and happiness after talking about their problems:

- *"She felt she was part of it and had something in common with the others, even though she is usually not a joiner."*
- *"It made him feel important—like he was a leader in opening up."*
- *"She thought she was the leader of the group members."*
- *"Before meetings, he was high-spirited and excited to come. I [his wife] tended to forget the meeting was coming more than he did—he never forgot. He looked forward to it and made his own transportation arrangements."*
- *"She was reluctant to go at first. Then, eager from then on. She practically left me [her husband] before getting to the meeting room."*
- *"He felt calm and upbeat after the meetings. He said beautiful and profound things to me [his wife] at these times—he was very open emotionally."*

Caregivers all thought their relatives' lives had changed as a result of the group; specifically, patients feeling more reassured, calmer, and more open about Alzheimer's disease:

- *"Recently, he talked with our houseguests about Alzheimer's disease—this was unusual."*
- *"He feels less alone. He's accepted having the illness and his understanding of the illness increased with the group."*

Caregivers felt the group helped the patients by "normalizing" their experience, improving mood, and adding organization to the patient's life.

- *"He felt safe to express his concerns and accepted by others. He realized he wasn't the only one and wasn't even as bad off as he thought."*
- *"She did talk about the group after it ended and up to 3 weeks later."*
- *"There's more verbal exchange between us [wife and me] now."*
- *"It gave him a purpose and some structure."*
- *"It helped him identify the cause of his behavior. He's a little more comfortable with the illness—he had support while coming to terms with it."*

None of the caregivers had any concerns about how the patients responded, and all wanted their relatives to continue attending a group. Caregivers expressed appreciation for the patients' experiences and surprise and frustration that other services were not available locally. One caregiver regretted that this group experience had not been possible even sooner in the course of the illness.

DISCUSSION

This study established that patients with early-stage dementia who had been given a diagnosis of Alzheimer's dis-

ease had responses and concerns
that they could express in interviews and in a support group. Comparison between treatment and control participants did not show
statistically significant differences
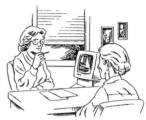
or changes over time in outcome measures. However, few
existing assessment instruments are sensitive enough to
make distinctions specific to mild dementia or the early
stages of caregiving. Data from supplemental clinical interviews do suggest that the patients and caregivers perceived multiple benefits from the intervention that may
have affected their well-being. The study describes some
of the issues unique to the early stages of Alzheimer's disease and demonstrates positive reactions to a particular
service approach, which suggests that patient support
groups are warranted, feasible, and potentially therapeutic
at this point in the disease course.

There are several limitations in this research. Study
results apply only to those who met the inclusion criteria.
Limited time and resources made it impossible to measure long-term effects of the intervention. The pilot nature of the project necessitated a small sample size and
scope. Furthermore, the occurrence of other events that
created additional stresses in the lives of the patients and
caregivers (e.g., deaths of friends) made it difficult to iso-
late the impact of this intervention alone.

Replication can be undertaken to determine effectiveness through larger studies with longer-term follow-up.
Assessment instruments and outcome measures sensitive
to the diversity of patients with mild dementia and their
caregivers in terms of specific impairments, acceptance of
the illness, and adjustments required might be developed
and standardized.

Further research paralleling service expansion is encouraged because it is obvious that patients with early dementia have many issues to discuss when given the opportunity. Patients in this study were articulate, attentive, insightful, and empathic in the group setting, and experienced great relief in talking with others who had similar problems. Therefore, the need for and potential benefits of group support appear to be analogous to those of caregivers and individuals with other common problems.

Group process issues are unique with the dementia population, though, requiring facilitation techniques that accommodate the patients' cognitive impairments and emotional reactions. Well-qualified facilitators and careful screening of participants for mild memory loss, openness about diagnosis, and appropriate communication and social skills will maximize the chances that patients have the desire and ability to discuss their concerns about Alzheimer's disease and value the chance to do so.

CONCLUSION

Patients with early dementia who seek information and support after being diagnosed with Alzheimer's disease historically have had few places to turn for follow-up. Although patients with Alzheimer's disease have typically been dehumanized and regarded as unable to express their thoughts and emotions, subjects in this study described a sense of success and satisfaction from their participation. Professionals who assume there is little they can do for patients with Alzheimer's disease may not realize how much the patients can accomplish for themselves. Although it is challenging to be asked difficult, pointed questions about the illness, the window of time during which those who have it can act on information received is poignantly narrow. The longer they must wait for support groups to be available, the less likely it is that they will have the opportunity to experience one.

Thus, there is a sense of urgency about the need for ongoing work in this area, and much that can and must be done. The intervention could be varied in length, size, and format and modified to serve distinct subpopulations, such as patients of a specific age range, gender, or culture. The development and evaluation of other program components, such as concurrent or conjoint groups for caregivers, are extremely important. In addition, written materials that remind patients, families, and professionals of the wellness (as well as the dysfunction) inherent in the early stages of dementia could serve an essential educational purpose.

Service providers across and outside of the United States are increasingly aware of these unmet needs, and many are beginning implementation efforts. Although support groups cannot reverse or halt disease progression, they may help patients and their families understand the illness, address their concerns, and learn about other resources available to them. It is hoped that the findings presented in this research study advocate strongly for initiation of public policy, continued research, and expanded program development to create a new starting point on the continuum of dementia care.

BIBLIOGRAPHY

Advisory Panel on Alzheimer's Disease. (1991). *Third report of the advisory panel on Alzheimer's disease.* Washington, DC: U.S. Department of Health & Human Services.

Akerlund, B.M., & Norberg, A. (1986). Group psychotherapy with demented patients. *Geriatric Nursing, 7,* 83–84.

American Psychiatric Association. (1994). *Diagnostic and statistical manual of mental disorders* (4th ed.). Washington, DC: Author.

Aronson, Miriam K. (Ed.). (1988). *Understanding Alzheimer's disease.* New York: Charles Scribner's Sons.

Austrom, M.G., & Hendrie, H.C. (1990, March/April). Death of the personality: The grief response of the Alzheimer's disease family caregiver. *The American Journal of Alzheimer's Care and Related Disorders and Research,* 16–27.

Bailey, E. (1989, March/April). Red on your head: Communicating in the here and now with Alzheimer's patients. *The American Journal of Alzheimer's Care and Related Disorders and Research,* 24–27.

Barnes, R.F., Raskind, M.A., Scott, M., & Murphy, C. (1981). Problems of families caring for Alzheimer patients: Use of a support group. *Journal of the American Geriatrics Society, 29*(2), 80–85.

Butler, R., & Lewis, M. (1991). *Aging and mental health: Positive psychosocial and biomedical approaches* (4th ed.). New York: Macmillan.

Cohen, D. (1991, May/June). The subjective experience of Alzheimer's disease: The anatomy of an illness as perceived by patients and families. *The American Journal of Alzheimer's Care and Related Disorders and Research,* 6–11.

Cohen, D., & Eisdorfer, C. (1986). *The loss of self: A family resource for the care of Alzheimer's disease and related disorders.* New York: Norton.

Cohen, G. (1988). One psychiatrist's view. In L. Jarvik &

C. Winograd (Eds.), *Treatments for the Alzheimer's patient: The long haul* (pp. 96–104). New York: Springer.

Cotrell, V., & Lein, L. (1993). Awareness and denial in the Alzheimer's disease victim. *Journal of Gerontological Social Work, 19*(3/4), 115–132.

Cotrell, V., & Schulz, R. (1993). The perspective of the patient with Alzheimer's disease: A neglected dimension of dementia research. *The Gerontologist, 33*(2), 205–211.

David, P. (1991, July/August). Effectiveness of group work with the cognitively impaired older adult. *The American Journal of Alzheimer's Care and Related Disorders and Research,* 10–16.

Drickamer, M.A., & Lachs, M.S. (1992). Should patients with Alzheimer's disease be told their diagnosis? *The New England Journal of Medicine, 326*(14), 947–951.

Dubler, N. (1982). A legal view: The patient's and family's right to know. *Generations, 7*(1), 11–13.

Erde, E., Nadal, E., & Scholl, T. (1988). On truth telling and the diagnosis of Alzheimer's disease. *The Journal of Family Practice, 26*(4), 401–406.

Folstein, M.F., Folstein, S.E., & McHugh, P.R. (1975). Minimental state: A practical method for grading the cognitive state of patients for the clinician. *Journal of Psychiatric Research, 12,* 189–198.

George, L. (1989). Services research: Research problems and possibilities. In E. Light & B. Lebowitz (Eds.), *Alzheimer's disease treatment and family stress: Directions for research* (pp. 401–433). Rockville, MD: U.S. Department of Health & Human Services.

Goldstein, M.K., Gwyther, L.P., Lazaroff, A.E., & Thal, L.J. (1991). Managing early Alzheimer's disease. *Patient Care, 25,* 44–70.

Gonyea, J. (1989). Alzheimer's disease support groups: An analysis of their structure, format and perceived benefits. *Social Work in Health Care, 14*(1), 61–73.

Gonyea, J., & Silverstein, N. (1991). The role of Alzheimer's disease support groups in families' utilization of community services. *Journal of Gerontological Social Work, 16*(3/4), 43–55.

Gwyther, L., & Blazer, D. (1984). Family therapy and the dementia patient. *American Family Physician, 29*(5), 149–156.

Gwyther, L., & Brooks, B. (1984). *Mobilizing networks of mutual support: How to develop Alzheimer's caregivers' support groups*. Durham, NC: Duke Family Support Program, Duke University Medical Center.

Hamilton, M. (1960). A Rating Scale for Depression. *Journal of Neurology, Neurosurgery, and Psychiatry, 23*, 56–62.

Kubler-Ross, E. (1969). *On death and dying*. New York: Macmillan.

Linn, M.W., Sculthorpe, W.B., Evje, M., Slater, P.H., & Goodman, S.P. (1969). A Social Dysfunction Rating Scale. *Journal of Psychiatric Research, 6*, 299–306.

Lipkowitz, R. (1982). Research builds esteem: A model patient/family group program. *Generations, 7*(1), 42–43.

McAfee, M., Ruh, P., Bell, P., & Martichuski, D. (1989). Including persons with early stage Alzheimer's disease in support groups and strategy planning. *The American Journal of Alzheimer's Care and Related Disorders and Research, 4*(6), 18–22.

Miller, M.D. (1989). Opportunities for psychotherapy in the management of dementia. *Journal of Geriatric Psychiatry and Neurology, 2*(1), 11–17.

Oppenheim, G. (1994). The earliest signs of Alzheimer's disease. *Journal of Geriatric Psychiatry and Neurology, 7*(2), 116–120.

Pearlin, L.I., Mullan, J.T., Semple, S.J., & Skaff, M.M. (1990). Caregiving and the stress process: An overview of concepts and their measures. *The Gerontologist, 30*(5), 583–591.

Pearson, J.L., Teri, L., Reifler, B.V., & Raskind, M.A. (1989). Functional status and cognitive impairment in Alzheimer's patients with and without depression. *Journal of the American Geriatrics Society, 37*, 1117–1121.

Quayhagen, M., & Quayhagen, M. (1989). Differential effects of family-based strategies on Alzheimer's disease. *The Gerontologist, 29*, 150–155.

Rabins, P., Mace, N., & Lucas, M. (1982). The impact of dementia on the family. *Journal of the American Medical Association, 248*, 333–335.

Reisberg, B., Ferris, S.H., de Leon, M.J., & Crook, T. (1982). The Global Deterioration Scale for assessment of primary dementia. *American Journal of Psychiatry, 139*, 1136–1139.

Sabat, S. (1994, May/June). Recognizing and working with remaining abilities: Toward improving the care of Alzheimer's disease sufferers. *The American Journal of Alzheimer's Care and Related Disorders and Research,* 8–16.

Sadavoy, J., & Robinson, A. (1989). Psychotherapy and the cognitively-impaired elderly. In D.K. Conn, A. Grek, & J. Sadavoy (Eds.), *Psychiatric consequences of brain disease in the elderly* (pp. 101–135). New York: Plenum.

Schmall, V. (1984, Winter). What makes a support group good? It doesn't just happen. *Generations,* 64–67.

Teri, L., Hughes, J.P., & Larson, E.B. (1990). Cognitive deterioration in Alzheimer's disease: Behavioral and health factors. *Journal of Gerontology: Psychological,* 45(2), 58–63.

Thompson, L., Wagner, B., Zeiss, A., & Gallagher, D. (1989). Cognitive/behavioral therapy with early stage Alzheimer's patients: An exploratory view of the utility of this approach. In E. Light & B. Lebowitz (Eds.), *Alzheimer's disease treatment and family stress: Directions for research* (pp. 383–397). Washington, DC: U.S. Government Printing Office.

U.S. Congress, Office of Technology Assessment.(1987). *Losing a million minds.* Washington, DC: U.S. Government Printing Office.

U.S. Congress, Office of Technology Assessment. (1990). *Confused minds, burdened families: Finding help for people with Alzheimer's and other dementias.* Washington, DC: U.S. Government Printing Office.

U.S. Department of Health and Human Services. (1994). *Seventh report of the Council on Alzheimer's Disease Progress in Research.* Washington, DC: Author.

Van Wylen, M., & Dykema-Lamse, J. (1990) Feelings group for adult day care. *The Gerontologist,* 30(4), 557–559.

Williams, D., Vitiello, M., Ries, R., Bokan, J., & Prinz, P. (1988). Successful recruitment of elderly community-dwelling subjects for Alzheimer's disease research. *Journal of Gerontology: Medical Sciences,* 43, M69–M74.

Yale, R. (1989). Support groups for newly diagnosed Alzheimer's clients. *Clinical Gerontologist,* 8(3), 86–89.

Yale, R. (1991). *A guide to facilitating support groups for newly diagnosed Alzheimer's patients.* Los Altos: Alzheimer's Association, Greater San Francisco Bay Area Chapter.

Yalom, I. (1975). *The theory and practice of group psychotherapy* (2nd ed.). New York: Basic Books.

INDEX

Page numbers followed by "f" indicate figures; those followed by "t" indicate tables.